OXFORD MEDICAL PUBLICATIONS

ICHPPC-2

ICHPPC-2

International Classification of Health Problems in Primary Care (1979 Revision)

An adaptation of the *International Classification of Diseases* (*9th revision*), intended for use in General Medicine (*ICD-9-GM*).

Prepared by the Classification Committee of WONCA (World Organization of National Colleges, Academies, and Academic Associations of General Practitioners/Family Physicians) in collaboration with the World Health Organization.

Oxford New York Toronto
OXFORD UNIVERSITY PRESS
1979

Oxford University Press, Walton Street, Oxford OX2 6DP

Oxford London Glasgow
New York Toronto Melbourne Wellington
Kuala Lumpur Singapore Jakarta Hong Kong Tokyo
Delhi Bombay Calcutta Madras Karachi
Nairobi Dar Es Salaam Cape Town

© *WONCA, 1979*

British Library Cataloguing in Publication Data
World Organisation of National Colleges, Academies
and Academic Associations of General Practitioners/
Family Physicians. *Classification Committee*
International classification of health problems in
primary care. – 1979 revision. – (Oxford medical
publications).
1. Nosology
I. Title   II. World Health Organization.
International classification of diseases
III. Series
616'.001'2   RB115   79–40153

ISBN 0-19-261186-0
ISBN 0-19-261195-X Pbk

Text set in 11/12 pt Photon Times, printed and bound in Great Britain at The Pitman Press, Bath

Contents

Introduction 1

There can be little doubt about the scientific importance of ICHPPC: since the introduction of the first version in 1975, it has become the benchmark for the study of expressed morbidity and workload in Family/General Practice. It has been translated into six languages and is used by family practice recorders all over the world. But ICHPPC also has a wider symbolic importance, something which should be considered by all family doctors, even those whose interests lie outside research.

Before 1972 the idea of one uniform classification of the problems which constitute the daily work of family physicians everywhere was a dream without a substance. Workers in several countries had developed the theoretical basis of primary care classification, and classifications for local use had been devised and used; but until they talked to each other, these workers were unaware that they had all come to very similar conclusions. The WONCA World Conference in Melbourne was the catalyst: since then the taxonomy of primary care has never looked back.

Incredible though it may seem, the lengthy and detailed work of devising a classification, of debating each rubric, of testing it in nine countries, of revising it, and preparing it for publication, was accomplished almost entirely by mail. The Committee only met at WONCA Conferences for a few days every two years to debate the most contentious issues, and to renew the sense of friendship and unity-of-purpose which was the motivating force behind their work.

It seems that the ingredients for this sort of advance in Family Medicine are these: a group of enthusiastic family doctors from various countries, who share a special interest and who meet from time to time in circumstances which allow them to become friends, are able to tell others what they have learned from their work, listen carefully to differing points of view, and resolve differences comfortably and without rancour. It is a winning formula, one which holds the promise of great things to come for Family Medicine. Letting this sort of thing happen is the main function of WONCA.

ICHPPC is a specific proof-positive example of the type of scientific contribution that WONCA is capable of. Perhaps, even more important, is that the use of ICHPPC will definitely influence the quality and better understanding of health care as provided by the family physicians of the world.

I strongly recommend that all family physicians and primary care providers familiarize themselves with this most important instrument of health care and make a proper use of it.

Edward J. Kowalewski, M.D.

President, The World Organization of National Colleges, Academies, and Academic Associations of General Practice/Family Medicine

Introduction 2

The *International Classification of Diseases, Ninth Revision (ICD-9)*, is the latest version of a classification that originated as the International List of Causes of Deaths, adopted in 1893 by the International Statistical Institute. The classification was revised at ten-yearly intervals and at the Sixth Revision in 1948, the first undertaken by the World Health Organization, its scope was extended to include non-fatal conditions and its use was recommended for morbidity statistics as well as for mortality. Subsequent revisions have enhanced its usefulness for morbidity applications by increasing the specificity of rubrics and by emphasizing manifestations of disease rather than aetiology.

A number of adaptations of the ICD to particular specialties have been prepared or are projected. Already published are the *Application of the ICD to Dentistry and Stomatology (ICD-DA)* and the *International Classification of Diseases for Oncology (ICD-O)*; in preparation are adaptations for ophthalmology, pediatrics, and dermatology. All these specialist adaptations provide additional detail by means of further subdivision of the relevant ICD rubrics. *ICHPPC-2*, on the other hand, is rather a 'generalist' adaptation that groups the detailed ICD rubrics into a shorter list of conditions significant in primary medical care.

ICHPPC-2 is much closer to *ICD-9* than was *ICHPPC-1* to *ICD-8* and there are now only a few instances where an ICD rubric is split between two ICHPPC groups. Correspondence between the two classifications is, therefore, almost complete. I am happy to welcome *ICHPPC-2* into the growing family of ICD adaptations under its other title of *ICD-9-GM* (an adaptation of the International Classification of Diseases, Ninth Revision, intended for use in General Medicine).

Karel Kupka, M.D.
Chief Medical Officer, International Classification of Diseases, World Health Organization

Introduction 3

In 1958 a report of studies conducted by members of the (now Royal) College of General Practitioners in the United Kingdom demonstrated that almost half the problems brought to family physicians could not be assigned a 'diagnosis', at least at the initial visit, that was compatible with the rubrics of the World Health Organization's *International Classification of Diseases* (ICD). Over the next few years a group of the College's members evolved a classification of symptoms, complaints, conditions, problems, and reasons for seeking help that reflected the array of perceived illness and other aberrations of living that constitute the burden of suffering at the level of primary care. This new classification was materially different both in concept and terminology from the traditional ICD which largely classified causes of death. Over the years the RCGP's classification was refined and expanded. It was field-tested in many countries and further modified in the early seventies by an international Classification Committee established by the World Organization of National Colleges, Academies, and Academic Associations of General Practitioners/Family Physicians (WONCA). The labors of this group produced the International Classification of Health Problems in Primary Care (ICHPPC); it was officially adopted by WONCA in 1974 and published by the American Hospital Association and the Royal College of General Practitioners in 1975.

The rapid adoption of ICHPPC by practitioners in many countries was accompanied by concern that it be made completely compatible with the Ninth Revision of the ICD to be introduced throughout the world in January 1979. Fruitful negotiations with the authorities of the World Health Organization resulted in formal endorsement of the ICHPPC concept. Rapid and energetic work by current members of the WONCA Classification Committee and technical assistance provided by the staff of the World Health Organization in Geneva and its North American Center for Disease Classification at the National Center for Health Statistics in Washington DC has resulted in this major revision. Based on further field-testing, the present version is almost completely compatible with *ICD-9*.

After taking careful note of the diversity of terms used to describe that level of formal medical care that underpins any health-care enterprise, the new classification has been assigned the term 'General Medicine' or *ICD-9-*

GM. Although health problems, practices, and systems differ around the world, and there may even be confusion in the terms used, such as primary care, general practice, family medicine, basic health services, and general medicine, there is broad agreement that a new classification for labelling the initial manifestations of disease brought to the primary levels of any formal health-care system was badly needed. This classification may not meet all the needs of developing countries and it falls short of providing a classification for many lay terms used to describe ill health, but it is a most important advance. At the least it is a concrete manifestation of the world-wide renaissance of primary care or general medicine which enables this aspect of illness and suffering that besets populations everywhere to be identified, classified, and counted more scientifically. In due course it should help policy-makers to set priorities and allocate resources in relationship to measures of need and expressed demand, and investigators to undertake research into the earliest manifestations of disease. As this body of knowledge grows it may modify our concepts of disease itself and this in turn may lead to other classifications. Indeed it seems probable that the tenth revision of the ICD may consist of a family of classification modules known generally as the International Classification of Health Problems and Diseases. It is a pleasure to congratulate all those responsible for this volume, which is only a beginning.

Kerr L. White, M.D.
Deputy Director, Division of Health Sciences, The Rockefeller Foundation, New York

Explanatory background

PURPOSE

ICHPPC is a grouping of those problems which comprise the content of primary medical care, so devised that valid, reliable statistical comparisons may be made between morbidity or workload reports from front-line medical practices anywhere in the world.

The following features of ICHPPC bore heavily on its design, its development and the organization for its maintenance:

a. ICHPPC represents a consensus on the content of primary care derived from the wide practical experience of many different family physicians from many countries.

b. Its broad-based input allows it to adapt readily to changes in concepts of health and disease, and to developments in primary care delivery.

c. The 'optional hierarchy' principle enables ICHPPC to accommodate the classification of problems of local importance and the special interests of recorders, without threatening comparability.

d. The full spectrum of first-contact medicine is covered: ICHPPC can be used comfortably by health-workers of various disciplines, in any setting from single-handed rural practice to the emergency department of a University hospital.

e. The brevity and simplicity of the list means that it is as effective for a secretary with pencil and paper as for a well-staffed medical records department with computer facilities.

f. While specifically directed towards the needs of primary care, *ICHPPC-2*, by virtue of its close alignment with the *International Classification of Diseases—ninth revision (ICD-9)*[1], allows comparisons with work from other fields of medicine.

HISTORY

The classification needs of primary care first came under consideration in the early 1950s as general practitioners began to record and study their daily work. It became a subject of major concern as multi-practice studies were initiated and the *Diagnostic Index (E-Book)*[2,3] made every GP into a potential recorder.

The first widely used classification for general practice was that of the British College of General Practitioners in 1959.[4] It went to three revisions and was used in many countries.

Meanwhile, family physicians in other parts of the world were discovering the need for a special classification of the problems of primary care;[5-13] they came to recognize certain underlying principles in the taxonomy of general practice; they devised classifications which were circulated (usually in mimeographed format), generally well-received, and widely used.

Many of these GP taxonomers came together in October 1972 at the Fifth World Conference on General Practice/Family Medicine in Melbourne, Australia. They agreed that there was a pressing need for one classification which could be accepted and understood by family physicians everywhere. This goal seemed to be attainable: roughly a third of all the rubrics in the classifications which were presented were common to every classification; everyone had reached the same conclusions about the underlying principles which would have to be followed.

Before this meeting ended, the World Organization of National Colleges, Academies, and Academic Associations of General Practitioners/Family Physicians (WONCA) had established a working party and charged it with the development of a tabular list to be based on the *International Classification of Diseases, eighth revision.*

The working party, later to become the WONCA Classification Committee, agreed upon a list, and field-tested it in over 300 practices in nine countries, for a total of more than 100 000 doctor–patient contacts. The rubric-by-rubric utilization figures and the comments and suggestions from this trial formed the basis on which the trial-version was modified to form *ICHPPC-1*.[14-16] On 7 November 1974, during the Sixth World Conference in Mexico City, that classification was unanimously accepted by the General Assembly of WONCA.

That first version of ICHPPC has now been revised to its present form, *ICHPPC-2*, in order to maintain comparability with the decennial revision of ICD, *ICD-9*.[1]

CHANGES FROM *ICHPPC-1*

Because only three years have elapsed since the publication of *ICHPPC-1*,[14] the Committee felt that no major changes in philosophy or content should be made in *ICHPPC-2*. The differences between this version and the last are due almost entirely to changes between *ICD-8* and *ICD-9*, which are themselves considered as being only intermediate in extent.[1]

The result of the revision is that 174 rubrics (48 per cent) are just the same in content and meaning as in *IPHPPC-1*, and only 111 (31 per cent) differ apart from minor changes in wording and layout. As explained below, the 'ICHPPC Code' may have changed even if the meaning of the rubric is identical: the 'Position Number', which is intended to be a relatively stable reference number, has rarely changed.

RELATIONSHIP OF *ICHPPC-2* TO *ICD-9*

The ninth revision of *ICD*[1] was intended to make the classification more useful for morbidity recording, moving away from its historic orientation towards the causes of death. There is considerable evidence of attention to the needs of ambulatory medicine in *ICD-9*, and indeed, despite the lack of direct representation by WONCA, it appears that *ICHPPC-1*[14] was considered, especially in the design of Section XVIII.

The result of these changes in ICD is that, although perfect conversion is not possible, *ICHPPC-2* is much more closely aligned to *ICD-9*, than *ICHPPC-1* was to *ICD-8*. In particular the number of ICHPPC rubrics that have a one-to-one relationship with a single ICD rubric (either at the third- or fourth-digit level) has increased from 145 to 160 (39 to 44 per cent).

More important still, the number of ICHPPC rubrics which consist (in whole or in part) of a split ICD rubric (at its most specific level) has declined from 114 to 27 (31 to 7 per cent).

For a little under half of the *ICHPPC-2* rubrics (48 per cent) comparability to *ICD-9* can be achieved by grouping together two or more rubrics of *ICD-9* (at the third- or fourth-digit level).

The Classification Committee would like to express its gratitude to Delray Green and Sue Meads from the North American Center for Disease Classification at the National Center for Health Statistics in Washington DC for their enormous help in the production of this new book.

MEMBERS OF THE WONCA CLASSIFICATION COMMITTEE

The following family physicians were involved in this revision of ICHPPC: Bent Guttorm Bentsen, Norway; Charles Bridges-Webb, Australia; Donald-Crombie, England; Boz Fehler, Republic of South Africa; Jack Froom, USA; Klaus-Dieter Haehn, West Germany; Bert Herries-Young, New Zealand; Poul Krogh-Jensen, Denmark; Henk Lamberts, Netherlands; Bill Patterson, Scotland; Kumar Rajakumar, Malaysia; Philip Sive, Israel; Gerhart Tutsch, Austria; Bob Westbury, Canada.

PLANS FOR THE FUTURE
Revisions

ICHPPC will be reviewed every four years, and will be revised at least every ten years to maintain its alignment with ICD.

Definitions

Work has begun on a companion volume of definitions for each rubric of *ICHPPC-2*, aimed at increasing the reliability of this classification. A nomenclature for family medicine may follow.

A special subcommittee will publish shortly a glossary of operational terms for General Practice/Family Medicine.

Long-term plans call for agreement on classifications for other facets of the primary care encounter:

a. the presenting complaints of the patient,
b. the reason for visit as interpreted by the provider,
c. the process—what the provider does for the patient,
d. the outcome of the encounter.

Translations

ICHPPC-2 will be made available in various languages besides English, as was the case with *ICHPPC-1*.

Clearinghouse

The Classification Committee are interested in receiving reports on the results of using ICHPPC, comments, questions, suggestions, and criticisms. Please write to the representative to the WONCA Classification Committee from your region, or to the Chairman of the Classification Committee, WONCA Secretariat, 50 Lambert Road, Royston Park, South Australia, Australia 5070.

REFERENCES

1. *International classification of diseases: manual of the international statistical classification of diseases, injuries and causes of death*, 9th revision: World Health Organization, Geneva (1977).
2. EIMERL, T. S. A practical approach to the problem of keeping records for research purposes in general practice. *J. R. Coll. Gen. Pract.* **3,** 246–52 (1960).
3. Research Unit of the Royal College of General Practitioners: the diagnostic index. *J. R. Coll. Gen. Pract.* **21,** 609–12 (1971).

4. Research Committee of the College of General Practitioners. 'A classification of disease.' *J. R. Coll. Gen. Pract.* **2**, 140–59 (1959).

5. WESTBURY, R. C. and TARRANT, M. Classification of disease in general practice: a comparative study. *Can. med. Assoc. J.* **101**, 82–7 (1969).

6. WESTBURY, R. C. The thorny road to an international classification of diseases in family medicine. *Fam. Physician Isr.* **4**, 214–19 (1974).

7. *Report on a National Morbidity Survey; Part 2.* National Health and Medical Research Council, Canberra (1969).

8. HUTCHINSON, J. M. The Australian morbidity survey, 1969–70. *Ann. Gen. Pract.* **16**, 68–72 (1971).

9. DREIBHOLZ, VON K. J. and ROHDE, P. A. Die Verdener Diagnosen-Liste. *Prakt. Arzt* **12**, 2–8 (1973).

10. FROOM, J. Classification of disease. *J. Fam. Pract.* **1**, 47–8 (1974).

11. LAMBERTS, H. De morbiditeitsanalyse—1972 door de groepspraktijk Ommoord. *Huisarts en Wetenschap* **17**, 455–73 (1974).

12. —— idem. *Huisarts en Wetenschap* **18**, 7–39 (1975).

13. —— idem. *Huisarts en Wetenschap* **18**, 61–73 (1975).

14. *International classification of health problems in primary care.* American Hospital Association, Chicago (1975).

15. FROOM, J. The International Classification of Health Problems in Primary Care. *Med. Care* **14**, 450–4 (1976).

16. LAMBERTS, H. De 'International Classification of Health Problems in Primary Care' en een nieuwe patientenkaart voor de huisartsgeneeskunde. *Huisarts en Wetenschap* **18**, 165–73 (1975).

Guidelines for the user

TABULAR LIST

Explanation of the columns (numbered from left to right)

Column 1

gives the 'Position Number'. In *ICHPPC-1*, these numbers ran straight through consecutively from 1 to 371. In *ICHPPC-2* they are not always in order, nine are missing altogether and seven new ones have been added; the reason for this rather awkward arrangement is to allow the position numbers of the first revision to be comparable to those in the original version; in broad terms any rubric bearing the same position number as before will contain the same problems as it did before. The nature and extent of any differences in meaning is indicated by the letter in Column 4 (see below).

If a rubric has been moved to a different position from that which it occupied in *ICHPPC-1*, it will appear in *parentheses* in Column 1 to make this clear.

As in *ICHPPC-1* there is a considerable amount of cross-referencing: terms cross-referenced away from their formal place carry no position number; in other words each position number appears only once.

Column 2

gives the four digit 'ICHPPC Code'. Once again most of the codes are identical to those in *ICHPPC-1*. If this *number* is different from the corresponding code number in *ICHPPC-1*, this is indicated by an *asterisk* to the left of the code number.

Notice that the ICHPPC Code is left-hand justified; if one of the three-digit code numbers is written or printed it must be followed by a character (a hyphen is used here, but any non-alphanumeric symbol will do) to move the number to the left.

Column 3

contains a description of each rubric, with inclusion and exclusion terms, and sometimes a short definition. Exclusion terms are followed by a reference to the appropriate ICHPPC Code.

Abbreviations and conventions

and   and, and/or

incl.   includes. This introduces some noteworthy problems which are found in this rubric.

excl.   excludes. This introduces some noteworthy problems which are *not* found in this rubric: they should be coded to the rubric shown in parentheses after each exclusion term.

NEC   Not elsewhere classified. When coding to a rubric containing this phrase, pause to consider whether the problem could be assigned to a more specific rubric.

NOS   Not otherwise specified. When coding to a rubric containing this phrase be sure that the diagnosis is expressed in non-specific terms which cannot be rendered more specific.

NYD   Not yet diagnosed. This is a subset of 'NOS'; the diagnosis is expressed in general terms because the diagnostic work-up is not complete.

Residual rubrics are found at the end of a section or subsection; their description includes the word '. . . other . . .'. Clearly 'NEC' is implied for all of the terms in these rubrics. A knowledge of the boundaries of the section or subsection is required; usually this will present no difficulty to physicians and experienced coders. If in doubt, consult the alphabetical list of *ICHPPC-2* or *ICD-9* (see below).

Section XVI: symptoms, signs, and ill-defined conditions. The phrases 'NEC', 'NOS', and 'NYD' could be applied to all the rubrics in this section, although they are not usually in the description. The rules for coding to these rubrics are the same as they would be if these phrases were included.

Spelling. For the sake of brevity, the American spelling convention has been adopted; thus: esophagus, edema, hemorrhoids, anemia, etc.

Punctuation has been held to a minimum for the sake of brevity and to assist machine processing.

Column 4

indicates whether there has been any change in the *content* of the rubric (as opposed to a change in one of the code numbers which label the rubric). If column 4 is empty, that rubric is exactly the same in *ICHPPC-2* as it was in *ICHPPC-1* (even though the Position Number or the ICHPPC Code, or both, may be different from those in *ICHPPC-1*). If there is a letter in column 4, there has been some change from the first version of ICHPPC;

the degree of change is indicated (on a subjective and approximate basis) as follows:

W   Minor change in Wording or structure of the rubric; the meaning and content of the rubric is unchanged.

L   There is a Lesser change in the meaning and content.

M   There is a Major change in the meaning and content.

N   This is a New rubric, not found at all in *ICHPPC-1*

Column 5

gives the equivalent codes in *ICD-9* (the ninth revision of the *International Classification of Diseases* published by the World Health Organization) for each rubric. 'ex.' indicates that the ICD codes which follow are not found in this rubric (e.g. in Position Number 25, '112(ex. 112.1, 112.2)' means that all of ICD code 112 except 112.1 and 112.2 is found in this rubric).

Those who are changing from ICHPPC-1 are advised first to look down Column 4 noting the nature and extent of the changes in meaning, and then to look down either Column 1 or 2—whichever code they use—to familiarize themselves with the new code numbers.

ALPHABETICAL INDEX

The basic arrangement of the alphabetical index is by underlying condition, with sites and other modifiers listed in alphabetic order under the lead term. Conditions expressed by adjectives appear in the list following the lead term. Each entry is accompanied by an ICHPPC code or by a cross-reference to another lead term. The code given in the alphabetic list should be checked in the tabular list to be sure that classification is correct. Remember that spelling is in the American convention: 'ae' and 'oe' are contracted to 'e'.

CONDENSED TITLES

Each rubric has been given a condensed title, consisting of 35 characters and spaces or less, designed for machine processing and computer printouts.

SOME ASSUMPTIONS

Multiple problems

It is assumed that users of *ICHPPC-2* will employ a recording system capable of documenting more than one problem at each visit. Studies have shown that most visits can be covered by recording three problems, and that more than six problems per contact is rare.

Parallel recording

ICHPPC was designed in the expectation that it would be used with a recording system equal or superior to the *E-book* (*Diagnostic Index*). This means that the diagnostic coding for each encounter should be accompanied by a code for:

a. the age of the patient,
b. the sex of the patient,
c. the status of each problem (e.g. new, recurrence, follow-up, modified diagnosis, previously diagnosed elsewhere, etc).

Type of coder

The classification is designed primarily for 'peripheral coding' (i.e. the health-care provider not only makes the diagnosis, but encodes it as well). Often data collection involves 'central coding' (i.e. the provider just names each problem in open language, leaving a secretary or record technician to provide the codes). Modifications have been made to ICHPPC in order to facilitate this approach, but coders who are used to other classifications may experience short-lived difficulty in getting the 'feel' of ICHPPC.

FAMILIARIZATION

New users are encouraged to begin by reading through the table of contents, the explanation of the tabular list and the list itself, so that they can appreciate the overall organization of ICHPPC and the pattern of individual rubrics. The axis of classification varies between aetiology, morphology, anatomical site, clinical manifestation, and symptom, as it does in ICD. In general terms infection, trauma, and symptoms tend to be grouped in their own special sections rather than according to their anatomical sites. Special attention should be directed to Sections V, XVI, and XVIII. Cross-references are used frequently to make the list easier to follow.

GENERAL RULES FOR CODING

The user should record and code every problem *actively coped with* at each contact. Background problems of which one is just passively aware should not be recorded. The user should code the *minimum number of rubrics* which *in his opinion* will *fully describe* the problems coped with. This judgement should be applied *at* (*or as of*) *the end of the encounter:* each problem should be entered at the *highest level of diagnostic refinement* of which the user can be *confident* at the time. For instance, if the clinical evidence cannot comfortably support a diagnosis of 'pneumonia', a lower level diagnosis such as 'cough' is preferable.

Users should code freely into the three classical areas of primary health care: *organic, psychological,* and *social.* For example 'cystitis' or even 'frequency of micturition' should not be entered if 'anxiety conversion' or 'mother-in-law problem' would be more appropriate. In most cases a *procedure* should be classified under the problem which necessitated it.

OPTIONAL HIERARCHY

Clearly no one international classification can fulfil every classification need for every user; inevitably users will sometimes want to separate out certain problems which are 'buried' in a rubric. If this problem arises, either because of increased incidence of a condition in one area or because of the special interests of the recorder, it can be solved easily, by assigning a special 'in-house' rubric to that condition. Provided that this rubric is put back into its original ICHPPC rubric when it comes to publishing the results, there will be no loss of the universal comparability which is the main purpose of ICHPPC.

CODING SYMBOLS

One of the unusual features of ICHPPC is that two codes are provided to identify the rubrics; each has certain advantages. The 'Position Number' consists of only three characters, a distinct advantage in cerebral and electronic data handling; it is designed to remain unchanged as ICHPPC is revised. The 'ICHPPC Code' closely approximates the ICD code (for 44 per cent of the rubrics it is identical) which is valuable in some circumstances, especially in jurisdictions where diagnostic data is required for billing.

Other coding systems have been suggested: in particular a mnemonic alphabetic system has been proposed which has great merit (it is obtainable through the WONCA Secretariat at the address given above). The user may use whatever system suits his needs best, provided that the content of each rubric is unchanged. It is the official policy of the Classification Committee that *Position Numbers* should always be used for the *publication* of results or *discussion* of ICHPPC.

PLACING AN OBSCURE PROBLEM

The procedure for coding a problem which cannot be found readily in the tabular list is as follows:

a. the condition should be sought in the alphabetical list of ICHPPC, looking for the underlying condition rather than a modifier (e.g. 'Reaction-drug' rather than 'Drug reaction'),
b. if it cannot be found there it should be sought in the alphabetical index (Volume II) of *ICD-9* and traced back to ICHPPC by searching column 5,
c. the appropriate rubric of *ICHPPC-2* should be examined to check that it is the correct position for the condition.

WRITE-INS

Users are advised to write down terms which are used locally, but which are not to be found in the tabular or alphabetical list. A synonym or closely related term in ICHPPC should be used for assigning the appropriate rubric, and the preferred term should be entered in the tabular or alphabetical list for future reference.

Quick guide to abbreviations

(A fuller explanation is found above)

Column 1	**Position Number**
( )	is out of sequence

Column 2	*ICHPPC Code*
*	*not* found in *ICHPPC-1*

Column 3	*Description of rubric*
and	and/or
excl.	excludes
incl.	includes
NEC	not elsewhere classified
NOS	not otherwise specified
NYD	not yet diagnosed

Column 4	*Comparison to ICHPPC-1:*
W	minor change in wording or structure of rubric; meaning the same
L	change in meaning or content of lesser degree
M	change in meaning or content of major degree
N	new rubric

Column 5	*Comparison to ICD-9*
ex.	excludes

Tabular classification of
health problems

Position no.	ICHPPC code	List of diseases, disorders, and health problems	Changes from ICHPPC-1	Comparable ICD-9 codes

I. INFECTIOUS & PARASITIC DISEASES

1	008-	**Intestinal disease of proven infective origin** *incl.* bacterial food poisoning, enteritis caused by a specified virus	M	001–008.6
2	009-	**Intestinal disease—presumed to be infec-tive, of either unspecified viral or unknown origin** *incl.* diarrhea presumed to be infective *excl.* diarrhea—*not* presumed to be infective, cause not yet determined & NOS (558-); vomiting, not presumed to be infective, cause not yet determined & NOS (7870); non-infective (specified) enteritis & gastroenteritis (558-); functional digestive disorders (558-, 5640, 579-); chemical-induced gastroenteritis (536-, 558-)	M	008.8, 009
4	011-	**Tuberculosis, all sites** *incl.* late-effects, recent positive conversion of TB skin test		010–018, 137
-		**Pleural effusion NOS (5119)**		
6	033-	**Whooping cough** *incl.* parapertussis & pertussis syndrome		033
7	034-	**Strep. throat (proven), scarlet fever, erysipelas**		034, 035
8	* 045-	**Poliomyelitis and other enterovirus diseases of central nervous system** *incl.* late effects, aseptic meningitis, slow virus infections	L	045–048, 138
9	052-	**Chickenpox**		052
10	053-	**Herpes zoster**		053
11	054-	**Herpes simplex, all sites**		054
12	055-	**Measles,** *incl.* complications *excl.* German measles (056-)		055
13	056-	**Rubella** *excl.* roseola infantum (057-)		056

Position no.	ICHPPC code	List of diseases, disorders, and health problems	Changes from ICHPPC-1	Comparable ICD-9 codes
14	057-	**Other viral exanthems** *incl.* pyrexia with rash NOS, roseola infantum		057
15	070	**Viral hepatitis** *incl.* all hepatitis presumed viral *excl.* hepatitis NOS (571-)	L	070
16	072-	**Mumps** *incl.* mumps orchitis		072
17	075-	**Infectious mononucleosis, glandular fever**		075
18	* 077-	**Conjunctivitis, presumed to be caused by a virus or chlamydiae** *incl.* viral pharyngoconjunctivitis *excl.* conjunctivitis NOS (3720)	L	077
19	* 0781	**Warts, all sites** *incl.* 'venereal' & plantar warts, verruca vulgaris, condyloma accuminata *excl.* seborrheic or senile (709-)	W	078.1
20	0799	**Viral infection unspecified** *excl.* influenza (487-)		079.9
21	084-	**Malaria**		084
22	090-	**Syphilis,** all sites & stages		090–097
23	098-	**Gonorrhea,** all sites		098
(372)	0994	**Non-specific urethritis** (i.e. urethritis apparently transmitted by intercourse which is not, or appears not to be, caused by the gonococcus) *excl.* other urethritis (597-)	N	099.4
24	110-	**Dermatophytosis & dermatomycosis** *incl.* athlete's foot, tinea, ringworm, onychomycosis		110, 111

Position no.	ICHPPC code	List of diseases, disorders, and health problems	Changes from ICHPPC-1	Comparable ICD-9 codes
25	112-	**Monilia infection, candidiasis, any sites except urogenital** *incl.* oral cavity, thrush, rectal mucosal candidiasis	W	112 (ex. 112.1, 112.2)
26	1121	**Urogenital candidiasis—proven** *incl.* monilial infection of vagina or cervix	W	112.1, 112.2
27	* 1310	**Urogenital trichomoniasis—proven** *excl.* leukorrhea NOS (629-)		131.0
28	127-	**Oxyuriasis, pinworms & all other helminthiases** *incl.* creeping eruption, trichiniasis, intestinal parasites NOS	W	120–129
29	132-	**Pediculosis & other skin infestations** *incl.* larvae, maggots, sand fleas, leeches	W	132, 134
30	133-	**Scabies & other acariases**		133
31	136-	**All other infective & parasitic diseases** *incl.* molluscum contagiosum, Vincent's angina, brucellosis, meningococcal infections, other venereal disease NEC, Reiter's disease, Coxsackie diseases, sarcoidosis, viral encephalitis, smallpox, cowpox, trachoma (see ICD for other inclusions)	W	020–027, 030–032, 036–041, 049–051, 060–066, 071, 073, 074, 076, 078 ex. 078.1, 079 ex. 079.9, 080–083, 085–088, 099 ex. 099.4, 100–104, 114–118, 130, 131 ex. 131.0, 135, 136, 139

Position no.	ICHPPC code	List of diseases, disorders, and health problems	Changes from ICHPPC-1	Comparable ICD-9 codes

II. NEOPLASMS

Malignant neoplasms

Position no.	ICHPPC code	List of diseases, disorders, and health problems	Changes from ICHPPC-1	Comparable ICD-9 codes
32	151-	Esophagus, stomach, large bowel, rectum, anus	W	150, 151, 153, 154
33	162-	Larynx, trachea, bronchus & lung		161, 162
34	173-	Skin, subcutaneous tissues *incl.* melanoma		172, 173
35	174-	Breast		174, 175
36	180-	Female genital tract *incl.* uterus, cervix (*incl. in-situ*), adnexa, vagina, vulva	W	179, 180, 182–184, 233.1
37	188-	Urinary & male genital tract *incl.* prostate, testis, bladder, kidney	W	185–189
38	201-	Hodgkin's disease, the lymphomata, the leukemias *incl.* multiple myeloma	L	200–208
39	199-	Other malignant neoplasms *incl.* secondary and metastatic neoplasms where primary site is unknown, carcinoma-*in-situ* (*excl.* carcinoma-*in-situ* of cervix: 180-), carcinoma of pancreas	W	140–149, 152, 155–160, 163–171, 181, 190–199, 230–232, 233 ex. 233.1, 234

Position no.	ICHPPC code	List of diseases, disorders, and health problems	Changes from ICHPPC-1	Comparable ICD-9 codes

Benign neoplasms

40	214-	**Lipoma, any site**		214
41	216-	**Skin** *incl.* mole, pigmented nevus *excl.* seborrheic (senile) warts (709-)	M	216
42	217-	**Breast** *excl.* simple cysts, chronic cystic disease (610-) skin of breast (216-)	W	217
43	218-	**Fibroids & others of uterus** *incl.* myoma, cervical polyp(adenomatous) *excl.* mucous cervical polyp (622-)		218, 219
44	* 228-	**Hemangioma, lymphangioma** *excl.* birth marks *incl.* angiomatous birthmarks (758-)		228
45	* 229-	**Other benign neoplasms** *incl.* those of brain, digestive system, endocrine system, large bowel, rectum, anal canal, and *incl.* polyposis of bowel, adenomatous cyst of ovary, adenomatous polyp of cervix *excl.* polyp of larynx or nose (519-), polyp of middle ear (388-), mucous polyp of cervix (622-), physiological cyst of ovary (629-)	W	210–213, 215, 220–227, 229

Unspecified neoplasms

46	239-	**Neoplasms, not yet determined whether benign or malignant** *incl.* polycythemia rubra vera *excl.* carcinomas-*in-situ* (180-, 199-) atypical or abnormal pap smear NOS (7950) mass, localized swelling (7822, 611-)	L	235–239

Position no.	ICHPPC code	List of diseases, disorders, and health problems	Changes from ICHPPC-1	Comparable ICD-9 codes

III. ENDOCRINE, NUTRITIONAL, & METABOLIC DISEASES AND IMMUNITY DISORDERS

47	240-	**Goitre & thyroid nodule without thyrotoxicosis** *excl.* proven neoplasm of thyroid (199-, 229-, 239-)	W	240, 241
48	242-	**Hyperthyroidism, thyrotoxicosis,** with or without goitre		242
49	244-	**Hypothyroidism, myxedema, cretinism**		243, 244
50	250-	**Diabetes mellitus** *excl.* hyperglycemia NOS; abnormal glucose tolerance test (7902)	W	250
-		**Abnormal unexplained biochemical test** *incl.* glucose tolerance test, multiphasic biochemical screening (7902)		
52	260-	**Vitamin deficiency, other nutritional deficiencies and disorders** *excl.* sprue, malabsorption syndrome (579-)	M	260–269
-		**Feeding problem (7833)**		
54	274-	**Gout** *excl.* pseudogout & crystal arthropathies (279-) hyperuricemia (7902)	M	274
55	* 278-	**Obesity**	W	278
56	272-	**Disorders of lipoid metabolism** (hyperlipidemia, abnormalities of lipoprotein levels, and raised levels of cholesterol & triglycerides) *incl.* congenital xanthoma	W	272
57	279-	**Other endocrine, nutritional & metabolic diseases and immunity disorders** *incl.* hypoglycemia, congenital metabolic disorders, thyroiditis, cystic fibrosis, disorders of fluids, electrolytes, or acid–base balance, fluid retention, amyloidosis, diabetes insipidus, hypopituitarism	W	245, 246, 251–259, 270, 271, 273, 275–277, 279

Position no.	ICHPPC code	List of diseases, disorders, and health problems	Changes from ICHPPC-1	Comparable ICD-9 codes

IV. DISEASES OF BLOOD & BLOOD-FORMING ORGANS

58	280-	**Iron deficiency anemia** *Excl.* in pregnancy, childbirth & puerperium (648-)	W	280
59	281-	**Pernicious anemia & other deficiency anemias** *incl.* folate deficient anemia *excl.* in pregnancy, childbirth & puerperium (648-)	W	281
60	282-	**Hereditary hemolytic anemias** *incl.* sickle-cell anemia, sickle-cell trait, thalassemia, spherocytosis		282
61	285-	**Other anemias** *incl.* anemia NOS *excl.* in pregnancy, childbirth & puerperium (648-)		283–285
62	287-	**Purpura, hemorrhagic conditions, coagulation defects, abnormality of platelets**	W	286, 287
63	2891	**Chronic & non-specific lymphadenitis** *incl.* mesenteric lymphadenitis, acute or chronic *excl.* acute lymphadenitis apart from mesenteric (683-), enlarged lymph node NOS (7856)		289.1–289.3
-		**Splenomegaly and/or hepatomegaly (7891)**		
-		**Leukemia, the reticuloses (201-)**		
-		**Polycythemia rubra vera (239-)**		

Position no.	ICHPPC code	List of diseases, disorders, and health problems	Changes from ICHPPC-1	Comparable ICD-9 codes

Abnormal hematological findings

64	* 288-	**Abnormal white cells** *incl.* leukocytosis, lymphocytosis, eosinophilia, agranulocytosis	M	288
-		**Abnormal platelets (287-)**		
-		**Raised ESR (7900)**		
-		**Abnormal red cells (7900)**		
-		**The anemias (280-, 281-, 282-, 285-) & in pregnancy (648-)**		
-		**Polycythemia (239-)**		
65	2899	**Other disorders of blood & blood-forming organs** *incl.* secondary polycythemia	L	289.0, 289.4–289.9

Position no.	ICHPPC code	List of diseases, disorders, and health problems	Changes from ICHPPC-1	Comparable ICD-9 codes

V. MENTAL DISORDERS

Psychoses (except alcohol & drug induced)

66	294-	**Organic psychosis** *incl.* non-alcoholic acute or chronic delirium, senile & presenile dementia	L	290, 293, 294
67	295-	**Schizophrenia, all types** *incl.* paranoid states & reactions		295, 297, 298.3, 298.4
68	296-	**The affective psychoses** *incl.* psychotic depression, involutional melancholia, mania, hypomania, manic-depressive, reactive depressive psychosis	L	296, 298.0, 298.1
69	298-	**Other & unspecified psychoses** *excl.* alcoholic (3031)	L	298.2, 298.8, 298.9, 299

Neuroses

70	3000	**Anxiety disorder, anxiety state** *excl.* anxiety causing a somatic complaint (3001)	W	300.0
71	3001	**Hysterical & hypochondriacal disorders** *incl.* factitious disorders, compensation neurosis, conversion hysteria, hysterical state, anxiety causing a somatic complaint, hyperventilation syndrome, cardiac neurosis *excl.* psychogenic disorders of sexual functions (3027), tension headache (3078), insomnia (3074)	W	300.1, 300.7, 306
72	3004	**Depressive disorder (neurotic depression)** *incl.* depression NOS, *excl.* brief depressive stress reactions (308-)	W	300.4, 311
73	3009	**Other neuroses** *incl.* neurasthenia, phobic state, obsessive compulsive disorders, occupational neurosis, neurosis NOS	W	300.2, 300.3, 300.5, 300.6, 300.8, 300.9

Position no.	ICHPPC code	List of diseases, disorders, and health problems	Changes from ICHPPC-1	Comparable ICD-9 codes

Other mental & psychological disorders

74	* 315-	Specific learning disturbance & delay in development of certain skills needed for schooling excl. mental retardation (317-)	W	315
75	* 3074	Insomnia & other sleep disorders	M	307.4
76	* 3078	Tension headache, psychogenic backache & other pain of mental origin (psychalgia) excl. headache NOS (7840), migraine (346-), lumbalgia (7242)	M	307.8
77	* 308-	Transient situational disturbance, acute stress reaction, adjustment reaction incl. grief reaction, bereavement, brief depressive reaction. May have additional code for cause (V602–V629)	L	308, 309
78	* 312-	Behaviour disorder (any age), disturbance of emotions specific to childhood & adolescence incl. hyperkinetic child, delinquency, kleptomania (any age) excl. character disorder (301-)	L	312–314
79	* 3027	Psychogenic disorder of sexual function incl. frigidity, impotence & loss of libido, psychogenic dyspareunia excl. marital problems (V611), vaginismus NOS & dyspareunia NOS in female (6250)	M	302.7
-		Other psychosomatic disorders of genito-urinary system (3001)		
80	3031	Chronic abuse of alcohol incl. alcoholism, alcoholic psychosis excl. non-dependent alcohol abuse (3050)		291, 303
81	* 3050	Acute alcohol intoxication, drunk, excessive alcohol intake NOS	W	305.0
82	* 3051	Abuse of tobacco		305.1
83	3048	Other drug abuse, habituation or addiction (incl. drug induced psychosis) incl. diazepam, cannabis, LSD, bar-biturates, laxatives, glue sniffing, etc.	W	292, 304, 305.2–305.9

Position no.	ICHPPC code	List of diseases, disorders, and health problems	Changes from ICHPPC-1	Comparable ICD-9 codes
84	301-	**Personality & character disorders**		301
85	* 317-	**Mental retardation**		317–319
86	* 316-	**Other mental & psychological disorders** *incl.* sexual deviation, tic, habit spasm, stammering & stuttering, anorexia nervosa, psychological causes of diseases classified elsewhere, psychological effects of head injuries *excl.* enuresis *not* clearly of psychological origin (7883)	W	302, ex 302.7, 307, ex 307.4, ex 307.8, 310, 316

Position no.	ICHPPC code	List of diseases, disorders, and health problems	Changes from ICHPPC-1	Comparable ICD-9 codes

VI DISEASES OF THE NERVOUS SYSTEM AND SENSE ORGANS

Diseases of the nervous system

87	340-	Multiple sclerosis		340
88	* 332-	Parkinsonism, paralysis agitans		332
89	345-	Epilepsy, all types *excl.* convulsions, febrile or NOS (7803)	W	345
90	346-	Migraine		346
-		Cerebrovascular disease, stroke (438-)		
-		Transient ischemic attack (435-)		
91	355-	Other diseases of the nervous system *incl.* cerebral palsy, meningitis NEC, Bell's palsy, trigeminal neuralgia, Morton's metatarsalgia, other peripheral neuropathy (primary or secondary), benign essential & familial tremor, reaction to lumbar puncture, restless legs syndrome *excl.* vertebrogenic compression syndromes (723-, 721-, 7244, etc.), post-stroke paralysis (438-), dementia (294-), effects of head injury on neurological (908-) or psychological (316-) function	L	320–331, 333–337, 341–344, 347–359

Position no.	ICHPPC code	List of diseases, disorders, and health problems	Changes from ICHPPC-1	Comparable ICD-9 codes

Diseases of the eye & adnexa

92	* 3720	**Conjunctivitis** *incl.* bacterial NOS, allergic *excl.* allergic with rhinorrhea (477-), conjunctivitis proven to be caused by specific organisms (in Section I), trachoma (136-), viral conjunctivitis (077-)	M	372.0–372.3
-		**Hay fever (allergic rhinitis) (477-)**		
93	* 3730	**Stye, hordoleum, chalazion, infected meibomian cyst, blepharitis**		373.0–373.2
94	* 367-	**Refractive errors** *excl.* blindness & reduced visual acuity NOS (369-)	M	367
-		**Corneal abrasion (918-)**		
-		**Foreign body in eye (930-)**		
96	* 366-	**Cataract**		366
-		**Blocked tear duct (in infants) (7436)**		
97	* 365-	**Glaucoma**		365
98	* 369-	**Blindness, reduced visual acuity** *excl.* snowblindness, night blindness (378-)	M	369
99	378-	**Other diseases of the eye** *incl.* retinal detachment, pinguecula, pterygium, retinopathies, iritis, keratitis, dacryocystitis, strabismus, red eye NOS, spontaneous subconjunctival hemorrhage, photophobia, tired eyes, diplopia, blurred vision, eye pain, arcus senilis, snowblindness, night blindness, ectropion, papilledema	M	360–364, 368, 370, 371, 372.4–372.9. 373.3–373.9, 374–379

Position no.	ICHPPC code	List of diseases, disorders, and health problems	Changes from ICHPPC-1	Comparable ICD-9 codes

Diseases of the ear & mastoid process

100	* 3801	Otitis externa *incl.* eczema of external auditory meatus *excl.* boil of external auditory meatus (680-)	W	380.1, 380.2
101	* 3820	Acute (suppurative) otitis media, acute myringitis, otitis media NOS	W	382.0, 382.4, 382.9, 384.0
102	3811	Non-suppurative otitis media acute or chronic	M	381.0–381.4
103	* 3815	Eustachian salpingitis or block	M	381.5, 381.6
104	* 386	Vertiginous syndromes, disorders of the labyrinth & vestibular system *incl.* labyrinthitis, Ménière's disease, benign paroxysmal & positional vertigo, vestibular neuronitis *excl.* giddiness, dizziness NOS (7804)	W	386
105	* 387-	Deafness NOS, otosclerosis *excl.* other specified causes of deafness (other rubrics in this section)	L	387, 389, 388.2
106	* 3804	Wax in the ear canal		380.4
-		Foreign body in ear canal (939-)		
107	* 388-	Other diseases of ear & mastoid process *incl.* ear pain NYD or NOS, chronic suppurative otitis media, mastoiditis, non-traumatic perforation of tympanic membrane, cholesteatoma, presbyacusis, acoustic trauma, tinnitus *excl.* deafness NOS (387-), traumatic perforation of tympanic membrane (889-)	M	380.0, 380.3, 380.5–380.9, 381.7–381.9, 382.1–382.3, 383, 384.1–384.9, 385, 388, ex. 388.2

Position no.	ICHPPC code	List of diseases, disorders, and health problems	Changes from ICHPPC-1	Comparable ICD-9 codes

VII. DISEASES OF THE CIRCULATORY SYSTEM

Diseases of the heart

108	390-	**Chronic rheumatic heart disease, acute rheumatic fever, Sydenham's chorea, with or without heart involvement** *excl.* chronic disease of valve or endocardium when not specified as rheumatic, and where rheumatic origin is *not* suggested on clinical grounds (e.g. it *would* be in the following: mitral stenosis, combined disease of mitral & aortic valves, tricuspid valve disease)	L	390–398
-		**Congenital anomalies of heart & circulatory system (746-)**		
109	410-	**Acute myocardial infarction, subacute ischemic heart disease**		410, 411
110	412-	**Chronic ischemic heart disease** *incl.* healed myocardial infarction, angina pectoris, asymptomatic ischemic heart disease, cardiosclerosis, aneurysm of heart *excl.* atherosclerotic valve disease (424-)	M	412–414
		Requires: additional code for any hypertension		
112	* 428-	**Heart failure, right-sided or left-sided**		428
		Requires: additional code for any hypertension or other known cause		
113	* 4273	**Atrial fibrillation or flutter**		427.3
114	* 4270	**Paroxysmal tachycardia** (supraventricular, ventricular, or unspecified) *excl.* tachycardia NOS (7889)	L	427.0–427.2

Position no	ICHPPC code	List of diseases, disorders, and health problems	Changes from ICHPPC-1	Comparable ICD-9 codes
115	* 4276	**Ectopic beat, all types** *incl.* PVB, PNB, PAB *excl.* wandering pacemaker (429-)		427.6
-		**Heart murmur NEC;** functional, innocent, not yet diagnosed (7852)		
-		**Cardiac neurosis (3001)**		
-		**Care of cardiac prosthetic device (V10-)**		
117	* 416-	**Pulmonary heart disease, (chronic) cor pulmonale**		416
-		**Abnormal ECG not classified elsewhere, unspecified abnormality of other tests of heart function (793-)**		
111	* 424-	**Disease of heart valve NOS, NYD, or specified as of non-rheumatic cause**	M	424
-		**Rheumatic valvular disease (390-)**		
118	429	**All other heart disease** *incl.* pericarditis (other than rheumatic), acute & subacute endocarditis, myocarditis, pericarditis, cardiomyopathy, heart block& other conduction disorders, cardiac arrest, other disturbances of heart rhythm, cardiomegaly	M	470–472, 476, 478, ex. pt. 478.1, 495, 500–510, 512–519

Blood-pressure problems

-		**Elevated blood pressure without a diagnosis of hypertension** (hyperpiesia) (7962)		
120	401-	**Uncomplicated hypertension, primary or secondary** *incl.* labile hypertension, hypertension NOS Requires: if secondary hypertension, code for underlying cause	M	401, pt. 405
121	* 402-	**Hypertension, primary or secondary with involvement of target organs** *incl.* involvement of heart, kidney or brain (Note: may code the effect as well)	W	401.0, 402–404, pt. 405, 437.2

Position no.	ICHPPC code	List of diseases, disorders, and health problems	Changes from ICHPPC-1	Comparable ICD-9 codes

Diseases of the vascular system

123	435-	**Transient cerebral ischemia** *incl.* transient ischemic attach (TIA)		435
124	438-	**Other cerebrovascular disease** *incl.* all types of stroke, subacute & chronic cerebrovascular disease, post-stroke paralysis		430–434, 436–438, ex. 437.2
125	440-	**Atherosclerosis except of heart, brain, gut or lung** *excl.* when causing arterial blockage (443-)	L	440
126	443-	**Other arterial obstruction & peripheral vascular disease** *incl.* intermittent claudication, other arterial blocks, Raynaud's phenomenon *excl.* aneurysm (459-), gangrene (7889-), chilblains (994-), blockage of: mesenteric arteries (579-), retinal artery (378-), renal arteries (598-), coronary arteries (410-, 412-), cerebral arteries (435-, 438-), pulmonary arteries (416-)	M	443, 444
127	* 415-	**Pulmonary embolism & infarction**		415
128	451-	**Phlebitis & thrombophlebitis** *incl.* phlebothrombosis, deep vein thrombosis, portal thrombosis *excl.* cerebral thrombosis (438-), phlebitis or thrombophlebitis in pregnancy (648-) or in puerperium (670-)		451–453
129	454-	**Varicose veins of legs, with or without ulcer or eczema** *incl.* venous stasis, venous insufficiency		454
130	455-	**Hemorrhoids** *incl.* thrombosed external piles (perianal hematoma), residual hemorrhoidal skin tags	W	455
131	4580	**Postural hypotension, low blood-pressure**		458
132	* 459-	**Other diseases of peripheral blood vessels** *incl.* aneurysm, polyarteritis nodosa, temporal arteritis, esophageal varices, varicocele, lymphangitis	W	441, 442, 446–448, 456, 457, 459

Position no.	ICHPPC code	List of diseases, disorders, and health problems	Changes from ICHPPC-1	Comparable ICD-9 codes

VIII. DISEASES OF THE RESPIRATORY SYSTEM

133	460-	**Upper respiratory tract infection, acute** *incl.* cold, rhinitis, nasopharyngitis, pharyngitis *excl.* that of proven specific origin (Section I)		460, 462, 465
134	461-	**Sinusitis, acute & chronic**		461, 473
135	463-	**Tonsillitis, acute, quinsy (peritonsillar abscess)** *excl.* that of proven streptococcal origin (034-)		463, 475
136	* 474-	**Hypertrophy & chronic infection of tonsils, and/or adenoids**		474
137	464-	**Laryngitis & tracheitis, acute** *incl.* croup, epiglottitis	W	464
138	466-	**Bronchitis, bronchiolitis, acute** *incl.* tracheobronchitis, bronchitis NOS	W	466, 490
139	* 487	**Influenza, without pneumonia** *excl.* gastric flu (009-), viral infection NOS (0799)	M	487, ex. 487.0
140	486-	**Pneumonia** *incl.* bacterial & viral pneumonia, influenzal pneumonia *excl.* aspiration pneumonia (519-)	M	480–486, 487.0
141	* 5110	**Pleurisy, all types except tuberculosis,** *excl.* pleurisy with effusion (5119) **Tuberculous pleurisy (011-)**		511.0–511.8
(5)	* 5119	**Pleural effusion NOS**		511.9
142	491-	**Chronic bronchitis** *incl.* bronchiectasis	M	491, 494
143	492-	**Emphysema, chronic obstructive pulmonary disease** (COPD, COLD) *excl.* bronchiectasis (491-)	M	492, 496
144	493-	**Asthma** **Hyperventilation syndrome, respiratory neurosis (3001)**		493
145	* 477-	**Hay fever, allergic rhinitis**		477

Position no.	ICHPPC code	List of diseases, disorders, and health problems	Changes from ICHPPC-1	Comparable ICD-9 codes
146	* 4781	**Boil or abscess in nose** *excl.* boil of skin of nose (680-)		pt. 478.1
-		**Foreign body in nose (939-)**		
147	519-	**Other diseases of respiratory system,** *incl.* deviated nasal septum, nasal polypi, chronic URTI, other diseases of larynx, allergic pneumonitis, pneumoconiosis, empyema, pneumothorax, lung complications of other diseases *excl.* cystic fibrosis affecting lungs (279-)	W	470–472, 476, 478, ex. pt. 478.1, 495, 500–510, 512–519

Position no.	ICHPPC code	List of diseases, disorders, and health problems	Changes from ICHPPC-1	Comparable ICD-9 codes

IX. DISEASES OF THE DIGESTIVE SYSTEM

148	520-	**Diseases of the teeth and supporting structures** *incl.* caries, dental abscess, teething, gingivitis, disorders of temporomandibular joint	W	520–526
149	528-	**Diseases of the mouth, tongue & salivary glands** *incl.* mucocele, apthous ulcer, angular cheilosis, effect of dentures, glossitis, stomatitis *excl.* Herpes simplex (054-)	W	527–529
150	530-	**Diseases of esophagus** *incl.* esophagitis *excl.* esophageal varices (459-)		530
151	532-	**Duodenal ulcer,** with or without complications		532
152	533-	**Other peptic ulcers** *incl.* gastric, gastrojejunal, marginal & peptic ulcer NOS		531, 533, 534
153	536-	**Disorders of stomach function and other diseases of stomach & duodenum** *incl.* indigestion NOS, dyspepsia, gastritis (incl. alcoholic), duodenitis *excl.* infective gastritis or duodenitis (008-, 009-)	W	535–537
-		**Vomiting, nausea NOS (7870)**		
154	540-	**Appendicitis, all types**		540–542
155	550-	**Inguinal hernia,** with or without obstruction		550
156	551-	**Hiatus hernia, diaphragmatic hernia**		551.3, 552.3, 553.3
157	553-	**Other abdominal hernias** *incl.* femoral, umbilical, incisional		551–553 ex. 551.3, 552.3, 553.3
158	562-	**Diverticular disease of intestines** *incl.* diverticulosis, diverticulitis		562

Position no.	ICHPPC code	List of diseases, disorders, and health problems	Changes from ICHPPC-1	Comparable ICD-9 codes
159	* 558-	**Irritable bowel syndrome (colospasm, spastic colon, mucous colitis) & other non-infective, non-ulcerative disorders of intestines** *incl.* allergic, dietetic & toxic gastroenteritis & colitis, diarrhea NOS presumed to be non-infective *excl.* intestinal disease which is either proven or presumed to be of infective origin (see Section I), regional enteritis (555-), vascular insufficiency of gut (579-), psychogenic diarrhea (3001-)	L	558, 564.1, 564.5
160	* 555-	**Chronic enteritis, ulcerative colitis, Crohn's disease**		555, 556
161	5640	**Constipation** *excl.* fecal impaction (579-)	W	564.0
162	565-	**Anal fissure and fistula, perianal abscess**		565, 566
163	* 5646	**Rectal & anal pain NOS** *incl.* anal spasm, proctalgia fugax, proctitis	N	564.6, pt. 569.4
164	* 5693	**Bleeding per rectum NOS** *excl.* (gastro)intestinal hemorrhage NOS (578-)	L	569.3
-		**Hemorrhoids (455-)**		
(276)	* 578-	**Hematemesis, melena** *incl.* (gastro)intestinal hemorrhage NOS	L	578
165	571-	**Cirrhosis & other liver diseases** *excl.* viral hepatitis (070-)	L	570–573
166	574-	**Cholecystitis, cholelithiasis, cholangitis, & other diseases of the gallbladder & biliary tract**		574–576
167	* 579-	**Other diseases of the digestive system** *incl.* mesenteric vascular insufficiency & block, intestinal obstruction, intussusception, ileus, dumping syndrome & other functional results of gastrointestinal surgery, secondary megacolon, diseases of pancreas, malabsorption syndrome, sprue, rectal polyp	W	543, 557, 560, 564.2–564.4, 564.7–564.9, 567, 568, 569 ex. 569.3, pt. 569.4, 577, 579

Position no.	ICHPPC code	List of diseases, disorders, and health problems	Changes from ICHPPC-1	Comparable ICD-9 codes

X. DISEASES OF THE GENITO-URINARY SYSTEM

Diseases of the urinary system

168	580-	**Glomerulonephritis, acute & chronic** *incl.* nephrosis		580–583
169	5901	**Pyelonephritis & pyelitis, acute** *incl.* kidney infection NOS *excl.* pyelonephritis, chronic (598-), in pregnancy, puerperium (6466)	L	590.1, 590.3, 590.8, 590.9
170	595-	**Cystitis & urinary infection NOS** *incl.* asymptomatic bacteriuria *excl.* in pregnancy, puerperium (6466)	M	595, 599.0
171	592-	**Urinary calculus,** all types & sites	W	592, 594
172	597-	**Urethritis (non-venereal) NEC, NOS** *incl.* meatitis, urethral syndrome	M	597
-		**Non-specific urethritis** (urethritis which is apparently transmitted through intercourse, and which is not, or appears not to be, of gonococcal origin) (0994)		
173	* 5936	**Orthostatic albuminuria** (postural proteinuria)		593.6
(373)	* 5997	**Hematuria NOS**	N	599.7
-		**Bacteriuria (595-)**		
-		**Other abnormal unexplained urine test NEC (791-)**		
174	* 598-	**Other diseases of the kidney, ureter, bladder, & urethra** *incl.* renal failure, chronic pyelonephritis, hydronephrosis, urethral stricture, urethral carbuncle	W	584–589, 590.0, 590.2, 591, 593 ex. 593.6, 596, 598, 599.1–599.6, 599.8–599.9

Diseases of the male genital organs

175	600-	**Benign prostatic hypertrophy** *incl.* hyperplasia, fibroma, median bar of prostate, prostatic obstruction NOS	W	600
176	601-	**Prostatitis, seminal vesiculitis**		601, 608.0
177	603-	**Hydrocele**		603

Position no.	ICHPPC code	List of diseases, disorders, and health problems	Changes from ICHPPC-1	Comparable ICD-9 codes

178	604-	**Orchitis, epididymitis** *excl.* mumps (072-), gonococcal (098-), tuberculous (011-)		604
179	605-	**Redundant prepuce, phimosis, balanitis**		605, 607.1
180	607-	**Other diseases of the male genitalia** *incl.* spermatocele, torsion of the testis	W	602, 607 ex. 607.1, 608 ex. 608.0

Diseases of the breast

| *181* | 610- | **Chronic cystic disease of the breast (fibroadenosis) & other benign mammary dysplasias** | W | 610 |
| *182* | 611- | **Other disorders of breast** *incl.* gynecomastia, non-puerperal breast abscess, fat necrosis, galactorrhea (not associated with childbirth), lump in breast NOS, mastodynia, nipple discharge | L | 611 |

Diseases of the female genital organs

183	* 614-	**Pelvic inflammatory disease** *incl.* salpingitis, oophoritis, endometritis *excl.* venereal diseases (090-, 098-, 136-)	L	614, 615
184	* 622-	**Cervicitis, cervical erosion and other abnormalities of cervix** *incl.* cervical leukoplakia, old laceration, mucous cervical polyp, cervical dysplasia *excl.* abnormalities of cervix in pregnancy, childbirth or puerperium (648-, 661-, 670-), adenomatous cervical polyp (218-), abnormal pap smear NOS (7950)	W	616.0, 622
185	* 6161	**Vaginitis NOS, vulvitis** *excl.* leukorrhea (non-infective), fluor vaginalis (629-), senile vaginitis (627-), proven specific causes (in Section I)	M	616.1
186	* 618-	**Uterovaginal prolapse** *incl.* cystocele, rectocele, stress incontinence NOS	L	618, 625.6

Position no.	ICHPPC code	List of diseases, disorders, and health problems	Changes from ICHPPC-1	Comparable ICD-9 codes
187	627	**Menopausal symptoms (climacteric)** *incl.* senile vaginitis, postmenopausal bleeding	M	627
188	* 6254	**Premenstrual tension syndromes**		625.4
(374)	* 6250	**Vaginismus, dyspareunia in the female** not specified as psychogenic	N	625.0, 625.1

Disorders of the menstrual cycle

189	6260	**Menstruation absent, scanty, or rare (amenorrhea, hypomenorrhea, oligomenorrhea)** *excl.* pregnancy (V223)		626.0, 626.1
190	6262	**Menstruation excessive (hypermenorrhea, menorrhagia), frequent (polymenorrhea) or irregular** *incl.* puberal bleeding, menometrorrhagia	M	626.2–626.4
191	* 6253	**Menstruation painful (dysmenorrhea) & intermenstrual pain (Mittelschmerz)**		625.2, 625.3
193	6269	**Intermenstrual bleeding & other disorders of the menstrual cycle** *incl.* metrorrhagia, ovulation bleeding, postcoital bleeding *excl.* postmenopausal bleeding (627-)	M	626.5–626.9
-		**Uterine fibroid (218-)**		
-		**Ovarian cyst——benign (229-),** **——malignant (180-),** **——physiological (629-)**		
-		**Pap smear——procedure (V70-),** **——abnormal (7950)**		
194	629-	**Other diseases of female genitalia** *incl.* Bartholin cyst or abscess, endometriosis, genital tract fistula, physiological ovarian cyst, leukorrhea, pelvic congestion syndrome	L	616.2–616.9, 617, 619–621, 623, 624, 625.5, 625.8, 625.9, 629

Position no.	ICHPPC code	List of diseases, disorders, and health problems	Changes from ICHPPC-1	Comparable ICD-9 codes

Fertility problems

| 195 | 606- | Sterility, reduced fertility of male or female | | 606, 628 |

Position no.	ICHPPC code	List of diseases, disorders, and health problems	Changes from ICHPPC-1	Comparable ICD-9 codes

XI. PREGNANCY, CHILDBIRTH, & THE PUERPERIUM

Position no.	ICHPPC code	List of diseases, disorders, and health problems	Changes from ICHPPC-1	Comparable ICD-9 codes
196	* 633-	**Ectopic pregnancy**		633
197	* 640-	**Bleeding during pregnancy** incl. antepartum hemorrhage—all causes, e.g. placenta previa, abruptio, threatened abortion		640, 641
198	* 6466	**Urinary infection in pregnancy or puerperium** incl. asymptomatic bacteriuria	W	646.5, 646.6
199	* 642-	**Toxemia, pre-eclampsia, & eclampsia of pregnancy, childbirth, & puerperium** incl. hypertension alone or with one other or more of the triad excl. edema, excess weight-gain, albuminuria as a complication of pregnancy, childbirth or the puerperium (648-)	M	642
200	* 636-	**Abortion, induced, legally or illegally** incl. any complications	M	635, 636
201	* 634-	**Abortion, spontaneous & NOS** incl. missed & incomplete & any complications		632, 634, 637
-		**Diagnosis of pregnancy (V223)**		
-		**Prenatal care (V220)**		
202	* 648-	**Other complications of pregnancy (prenatal)** incl. emesis & hyperemesis, false labor, post-term, edema and/ or albuminuria without hypertension, anemia; excl. complications of abortion	M	630, 631, 638, 639, 643–645, 646 (ex. 646.5, 646.6), 647, 648
203	650-	**Normal delivery**		650

Position no.	ICHPPC code	List of diseases, disorders, and health problems	Changes from ICHPPC-1	Comparable ICD-9 codes
204	661-	**Complicated delivery and some conditions (diagnosable either during labor & delivery, or before) which require special care to avoid complications in pregnancy, labor or delivery** (e.g. multiple pregnancy, fetal malposition, disproportion, large-for-dates, small-for-dates, elderly primipara, old Caesarian section, etc).	M	651–669
		Postnatal care (V24-)		
205	* 676-	**Mastitis, other disorders of the breast & nipple in the puerperium, and disorders of lactation** *incl.* suppression of lactation	L	675, 676
206	* 670-	**Other complications of puerperium (postnatal)** *incl.* infection of genital tract, postoperative complications of obstetrical surgery *excl.* urinary infection (6466), anemia (648-), toxemia syndromes (642-)	L	pt. 646.6, 670–674

Position no.	ICHPPC code	List of diseases, disorders, and health problems	Changes from ICHPPC-1	Comparable ICD-9 codes

XII. DISEASES OF THE SKIN & SUBCUTANEOUS TISSUE

207	**680-**	**Boil, carbuncle, cellulitis, abscess** *incl.* finger, toe, with or without lymphangitis *excl.* of: eyelid (3730), perianal (565-), ext. auditory canal (3801), male external genitalia (607-), female external genitalia (620-), inside nose (4781), infected surgical wound (998-), tissue of breast (611-, 676-), if also lymphadenitis (683-)	M	680–682
209	**683-**	**Lymphadenitis, acute** *incl.* abscess of lymph node *excl.* chronic lymphadenitis (2891), mesenteric lymphadenitis (2891), enlarged lymph node NOS (7856)		683
210	**684-**	**Impetigo** *incl.* secondary impetigo	W	684
-		**Erysipelas (034-)**		
211	**685-**	**Pilonidal cyst, fistula, pyoderma, pyogenic granuloma, infected sinus, ecthyma, & other infections of the skin & subcutaneous tissue**	W	685, 686
212	**690-**	**Seborrheic dermatitis & other erythematosquamous dermatoses** *incl.* dandruff		690
-		**Seborrheic (senile) warts (709-)**		
213	*** 6918**	**Atopic dermatitis or eczema** *incl.* infantile eczema & flexural dermatitis *excl.* diaper rash (6910)	W	691.8
214	**692-**	**Contact dermatitis & other eczema or dermatitis** *incl.* sunburn, due to cold, due to drugs taken internally, dermatitis NOS, eczema NOS *excl.* allergy NOS, allergic reaction NOS (9950), diaper rash (6910), rash NOS (7821)	M	692, 693

Position no.	ICHPPC code	List of diseases, disorders, and health problems	Changes from ICHPPC-1	Comparable ICD-9 codes
215	* 6910	Diaper rash (napkin rash)		691.0
-		Varicose eczema, varicose ulcer, stasis dermatitis (454-)		
216	6963	Pityriasis rosea		696.3
-		Purpura (287-)		
-		Dermatophytosis, dermatomycosis *incl.* athlete's foot, tinea (110-)		
-		Monilial skin infection (112-)		
217	6961	Poriasis with or without arthropathy		696.0, 696.1
218	698-	Pruritis & related conditions *incl.* lichen simplex chronicus, neurodermatitis, dermatitis factitia, anogenital pruritus, itch NOS		698
-		Herpes zoster (053-)		
-		Herpes simplex (054-)		
-		Pediculosis (132-)		
-		Scabies (133-)		
-		Molluscum contagiosum (136-)		
219	700	Corns, callosities		700
-		Warts, all sites, (0781)		
-		Mole, pigmented nevus (216-)		
-		Skin tumors: benign (216-), lipoma (214-), malignant (173-)		
220	7062	Sebaceous cyst *incl.* inclusion dermoid		706.2
221	703-	Ingrowing toenail, onychogryphosis, other diseases of nail		703
222	704-	Alopecia, folliculitis & other diseases of hair *incl.* sycosis barbae	W	704
223	705-	Pompholyx, other diseases of sweat glands *incl.* prickly heat, sweat rash, heat rash, dyshydrosis *excl.* hyperhidrosis (7808)	W	705
224	7061	Acne *excl.* acne-rosacea (709-)		706.0, 706.1

Position no.	ICHPPC code	List of diseases, disorders, and health problems	Changes from ICHPPC-1	Comparable ICD-9 codes
225	707-	**Chronic ulcer of skin** *incl.* bedsore *excl.* varicose ulcer (454-)		707
226	708-	**Urticaria** *excl.* angioedema, allergic edema (9950), drug allergy (9952), edema NOS (7823)	L	708
227	709-	**Other diseases of the skin & subcutaneous tissue** *incl.* erythema multiforme, erythema nodosum, rosacea, intertrigo, erythema NOS, lichen planus, ichthyosis, striae atrophicae, keloid, vitiligo, localized lupus erythematosis	W	694, 695, 696.2, 696.4–696.8, 697, 701, 702, 706.3–706.9, 709

XIII. DISEASES OF THE MUSCULOSKELETAL SYSTEM & CONNECTIVE TISSUE

Arthritis & arthrosis

Position no.	ICHPPC code	List of diseases, disorders, and health problems	Changes	ICD-9
228	* 714-	**Rheumatoid arthritis & allied conditions** *incl.* ankylosing spondylitis *excl.* psoriatic arthropathy (6961)	L	714, 720.0
229	* 715-	**Osteoarthritis (osteoarthrosis) & allied conditions** *excl.* of spine (721-)		715
230	* 7161	**Traumatic arthropathy (arthritis)** *excl.* effusion (7190), internal derangement of knee—acute (836-)—chronic (717-)	L	716.1
-		**Gout (274-)**		
288)	* 7194	**Pain in joint, arthralgia, stiffness in joint**	L	719.4, 719.5
289)	* 7190	**Swelling of joint, effusion of joint** with or without pain	W	719.0
231	* 725-	**Other types of arthritis & diffuse connective tissue disorders** *incl.* dermatomyositis, systemic lupus erythematosis, scleroderma (progressive), pyogenic arthritis, arthritis secondary to other diseases, the chondrocalcinoses, arthritis NYD or NOS, polymyalgia rheumatica, villonodular synovitis, palindromic rheumatism	L	710–713, 716 ex. 716.1, 719.2, 719.3, 725

Non-articular rheumatism

Position no.	ICHPPC code	List of diseases, disorders, and health problems	Changes	ICD-9
232	* 7260	**The shoulder syndromes** *incl.* rotator cuff syndrome, frozen shoulder, bursitis of shoulder, synovitis of shoulder, tendinitis around shoulder		726.0–726.2

Position no.	ICHPPC code	List of diseases, disorders, and health problems	Changes from ICHPPC-1	Comparable ICD-9 codes
233	* 7263	**Other bursitis, tendinitis, tenosynovitis, synovitis & peripheral enthesopathy** *incl.* synovial cyst, peritendinitis, bone spur, calcified tendon, tennis elbow *excl.* of shoulder (7260), ganglion (7274), bunion (736-), of spine (7242, 7244)	W	726.3–726.9, 727 (ex. 727.1, 727.4)
234	* 728-	**Other non-articular rheumatism and disorders of muscle, ligament, & fascia** *incl.* fibrositis, muscle pain, myalgia, myositis, panniculitis, fasciitis, Dupuytren's contracture, foreign-body granuloma *excl.* epidemic myositis (Bornholm disease) (136-)	W	728, 729 (ex. 729.5, 729.8)
(286)	7295	**Pain & other symptoms referable to limbs** *incl.* 'growing pains' in a child, leg cramps *excl.* from spine (7242, 7244), restless-legs syndrome (355-)	M	729.5, 729.8

Syndromes related to the vertebral column

Position no.	ICHPPC code	List of diseases, disorders, and health problems	Changes from ICHPPC-1	Comparable ICD-9 codes
235	* 723-	**Syndromes related to the cervical spine** *incl.* cervicalgia, cervical disc lesion, torticollis, cervicobrachial syndrome, radicular syndrome of upper limbs *excl.* osteoarthritis of spine (721-), cervical strain (8470), psychogenic tension headache (3078)		722.0, 722.4, 723
237	* 721-	**Osteoarthritis of spine** (any region) *incl.* spondylosis	M	721
238	* 7242	**Back pain (lumbar, thoracic, or sacroiliac) without radiating symptoms** *incl.* backache NOS, lumbalgia, lumbago, coccydynia *excl.* recent strain (8478), psychogenic backache (3078)	M	720.1–720.9, 724.1, 724.2, 724.5–724.9
239	* 7244	**Back pain (lumbar or thoracic) with radiating symptoms** *incl.* prolapsed or degenerated disc, sciatica *excl.* recent strain (8478), spondylolisthesis (758-)	M	722.1, 722.5, 724.3, 724.4

Position no.	ICHPPC code	List of diseases, disorders, and health problems	Changes from ICHPPC-1	Comparable ICD-9 codes
240	* 737-	**Acquired deformities of spine** *incl.* scoliosis, kyphosis, kyphoscoliosis, lordosis, curvature NOS *excl.* congenital deformities (758-), ankylosing spondylitis (714-)		737
-		**Paget's disease of the spine (739-)**		
-		**Scheuermann's disease (732-)**		
-		**Osteoporosis (7330)**		
-		**Tuberculosis of the spine (011-)**		
-		**Osteomyelitis (739-)**		

Other musculoskeletal & connective tissue disorders

241	* 7274	**Ganglion** of joint (capsule) & tendon (sheath)		727.4
242	* 732-	**Osgood–Schlatter's disease, other osteochondroses, & osteochondropathies** *incl.* Scheuermann's disease, Legg–Calve–Perthes disease, slipped femoral epiphysis, osteochondritis dissecans	L	732
243	* 7330	**Osteoporosis**		733.0
244	* 717-	**Chronic internal derangement of knee** *incl.* longstanding meniscus tear, loose body in knee, chondromalacia patellae *excl.* acute, current injury (836-), recurrent dislocation (739-)	L	717
245	* 736-	**Acquired deformities of limbs** *incl.* pes planus (flatfoot), hallux valgus-varus-rigidus, bunion, mallet finger, genu valgum-varum *excl.* congenital deformities & anomalies (754-, 758-)	W	727.1, 734–736

Position no.	ICHPPC code	List of diseases, disorders, and health problems	Changes from ICHPPC-1	Comparable ICD-9 codes
246	739-	**Other diseases of musculoskeletal system & connective tissue** *incl.* weakness in limb muscle or joint NOS, post-surgical back pain, osteomyelitis, Paget's disease of bone, costochondritis, arthrodesis, malunion or non-union of fracture, pathological fracture NOS, joint mice (excl. knee), recurrent dislocation *excl.* trigger finger (7663), curvature of spine (737-), late effects of polio (045-)	L	718, 719.1, 719.6–719.9, 722.2, 722.3, 722.6–722.9, 724.0, 730, 731, 733 ex. 733.0, 738, 739

Position no.	ICHPPC code	List of diseases, disorders, and health problems	Changes from ICHPPC-1	Comparable ICD-9 codes

XIV. CONGENITAL ANOMALIES

247	746-	**Congenital anomalies of heart & circulatory system**		745–747
248	754-	**Certain congenital anomalies of lower limb** *incl.* congenital dislocation of hip, genu recurvatum, bowing of long bones of leg, clubfoot—all types, & other congenital deformities of foot *excl.* pes planus (acquired) (736-)	M	754.3–754.7
249	* 7525	**Undescended testicle**		752.5
-		**Mole, pigmented nevus (216-)**		
-		**Hemangioma, lymphangioma (228-)**		
-		**Cretinism (244-)**		
251	* 7436	**Blocked tear duct, agenesis of lacrimal punctum**		pt. 743.6
252	758-	**Other congenital anomalies** *incl.* spondylolisthesis, spina bifida, cleft lip & palate, webbed fingers, Darwin's tubercle, tongue-tie, Meckel's diverticulum, congenital polycystic kidneys, birthmarks, supernumerary nipples *excl.* congenital metabolic disorders (e.g. cystic fibrosis) (Section III)	L	740–742, 743 (ex. pt. 743.6), 744, 748–751, 752 (ex. 752.5), 753, 754 (ex. 754.3–754.7), 755–759

Position no.	ICHPPC code	List of diseases, disorders, and health problems	Changes from ICHPPC-1	Comparable ICD-9 codes

XV. CERTAIN CONDITIONS ORIGINATING IN THE PERINATAL PERIOD

| 253 | 778- | **All perinatal morbidity & mortality conditions** | W | 760–779 |

incl. maternal conditions as they affect the fetus or newborn, factors in labor & delivery as they affect the fetus or newborn, dysmature or postmature newborn, one of multiple birth, respiratory distress syndrome, physiological jaundice, pneumonia, & diarrhea of newborn, umbilical sepsis, hemolytic disease of newborn, feeding problems in neonatal period *excl.* failure to thrive NOS (7834)

Position no.	ICHPPC code	List of diseases, disorders, and health problems	Changes from ICHPPC-1	Comparable ICD-9 codes

XVI. SYMPTOMS, SIGNS, & ILL-DEFINED CONDITIONS

Central nervous system & peripheral nerves

254	* 7803	**Convulsions** *incl.* febrile convulsions *excl.* convulsions in newborn (778-)	W	780.3
255	* 7810	**Abnormal involuntary movement** *incl.* tremor spasms, fasciculation *excl.* tic, habit spasm (316-), restless-legs syndrome (355-)		781.0
256	* 7804	**Dizziness, giddiness** *excl.* specific vertiginous syndromes (386-)	W	780.4
257	* 7845	**Disturbance of speech** *incl.* hoarseness *excl.* stammering, stuttering (316-)	M	784.3–784.5
258	* 7840	**Headache** *incl.* pain in head or face NOS *excl.* tension headache (3078), migraine (346-), atypical facial neuralgia (355-)	W	784.0
259	* 7820	**Disturbance of sensation, paraesthesiae** *excl.* restless legs syndrome (355-)		782.0

Eye

-		**Blurred vision (378-)**		
-		**Reduced visual acuity, blindness (369-)**		
-		**Refractive errors (367-)**		
-		**Eye pain, photophobia (378-)**		
-		**Red eye NOS (378-)**		
-		**Tired eyes (378-)**		
-		**Diplopia (378-)**		

Position no.	ICHPPC code	List of diseases, disorders, and health problems	Changes from ICHPPC-1	Comparable ICD-9 codes

Ear

-		Ear pain (388-)		
-		Deafness (387-)		
-		Tinnitus (388-)		

Cardiovascular & lymphatic systems

262	* **7865**	**Chest pain,** *incl.* precordial pain, painful respiration, pleurodynia, pleuritic pain	M	786.5
263	* **7851**	**Palpitation (aware of heartbeat)**		785.1
-		**Elevated blood-pressure not diagnosed as hypertension (7962)**		
264	* **7802**	**Syncope, faint, blackout**		780.2
(116)	**7852**	**Heart murmur NEC, or NYD;** functional, innocent		785.2, pt. 785.9
265	* **7823**	**Edema—localized or dependent** *excl.* fluid retention (279-), in pregnancy (648-), allergic (9950)	L	782.3
266	**7856**	**Enlarged lymph nodes, not infected** *incl.* lymphadenopathy *excl.* lymphadenitis—acute (683-), —chronic (2891)		785.6

Respiratory system

267	* **7847**	**Epistaxis**		784.7
268	* **7863**	**Hemoptysis**		786.3
269	* **7860**	**Dyspnea** *incl.* orthopnea, wheezing, stridor, tachypnea *excl.* hyperventilation of psychogenic origin (3001), respiratory distress of newborn (778-), respiratory failure (7889)	L	786.0, 786.1

Position no.	ICHPPC code	List of diseases, disorders, and health problems	Changes from ICHPPC-1	Comparable ICD-9 codes
270	* 7862	Cough		786.2
-		Hoarseness (7845)		
-		Painful respiration (7865)		
-		Pleural effusion—NOS (5119)—known cause—not TB (5110),—tuberculosis (011-)		

Gastro-intestinal system & abdomen

Position no.	ICHPPC code	List of diseases, disorders, and health problems	Changes from ICHPPC-1	Comparable ICD-9 codes
273	* 7830	Anorexia		783.0
274	* 7870	Nausea and/or vomiting *excl.* of pregnancy (648-), of newborn (778-)		787.0
275	* 7871	Heartburn		787.1
-		Indigestion (536-)		
-		Hematemesis, melena (578-)		
-		Bleeding per rectum NOS (5693)		
277	* 7891	Hepatomegaly and/or splenomegaly		789.1, 789.2
278	* 7873	Gas problems (wind) *incl.* eructation, bloating, gas gains in the adult, flatulence, passage of excess gas per rectum	W	787.3
279	* 7890	Abdominal pain *incl.* infantile colic		789.0
-		Rectal & anal pain (5646)		
-		Diarrhea NOS—presumed to be infective (009-),—presumed not to be infective (558-)		
-		Constipation (5640)		

Genito-urinary system

Position no.	ICHPPC code	List of diseases, disorders, and health problems	Changes from ICHPPC-1	Comparable ICD-9 codes
280	* 7881	Dysuria	L	788.1
281	* 7883	Enuresis, bedwetting, urinary incontinence *excl.* clearly of psychogenic origin (316-) Stress incontinence NOS (618-)	L	788.3

Position no.	ICHPPC code	List of diseases, disorders, and health problems	Changes from ICHPPC-1	Comparable ICD-9 codes
283	* 7884	Frequency of urination incl. polyuria, nocturia		788.4
-		Hematuria (5997)		
-		Bacteriuria (595-)		
-		Other abnormal urine findings (791-)		
-		Frigidity, impotence, reduced libido, psychogenic dyspareunia (3027)		
-		Dyspareunia NOS—female (6250), —male (607-)		
-		Vaginitis (6161)		
-		Breast pain (611-)		
-		Nipple discharge (611-)		
-		Breast lump (611-)		
-		Menses absent, scanty, or rare (6260)		
-		Menses excessive, frequent or irregular (6262)		
-		Menses painful (dysmenorrhea) or intermenstrual pain (6253)		
-		Menses otherwise abnormal, incl. intermenstrual bleeding, metrorrhagia (6269)		
-		Menometrorrhagia (6262)		
-		Menopausal symptoms (627-)		

Limbs & joints

-		Pain in limb incl. 'growing pains' in a child (7295)		
-		Leg cramps incl. nocturnal leg cramps (7295)		
-		Restless legs syndrome (355-)		
-		Myalgia, muscle pain (728-)		
-		Backache, lumbalgia (7242)		
-		Joint pain, arthralgia (7194)		
-		Swelling of joint (7190)		
-		Weakness in limb, muscle, or joint (739-)		

Position no.	ICHPPC code	List of diseases, disorders, and health problems	Changes from ICHPPC-1	Comparable JCD-9 codes

General signs & symptoms

290	* 7808	Excessive sweating, hyperhidrosis		780.8
291	* 7806	Fever of undetermined cause (pyrexia of unknown origin), hyperpyrexia		780.6
292	* 7821	Rash & other non-specific skin eruptions		782.1
-		Pruritis (698-)		
-		Allergy NOS (9950)		
-		Allergy to medications (9952)		
-		Contact dermatitis (692-)		
-		Atopic eczema, atopic dermatitis (6918)		
-		Urticaria (708-)		
		Allergic edema, angioneurotic edema (9950)		
-		Allergic reaction to insect bite or sting (910-)		
-		Allergic reaction to immunization (998-)		
-		Allergic reaction NOS (9950)		
-		Allergic rhinitis (477-)		
-		Allergic asthma (493-)		
-		Allergic gastro-enteritis or colitis (558-)		
-		Allergic conjunctivitis (3720)		
293	* 7832	Weight loss, cachexia	W	783.2, 799.4
294	* 7834	Lack of expected physiological development, failure to thrive		783.4
(53)	* 7833	Feeding problem: baby or elderly *excl.* feeding problem in neonatal period (778-)	L	783.3
-		Obesity (277-)		
295	* 7807	Malaise, debility, fatigue, tiredness *incl.* postviral syndromes *excl.* neurasthenia (3009)	L	780.7, 799.3

Position no.	ICHPPC code	List of diseases, disorders, and health problems	Changes from ICHPPC-1	Comparable ICD-9 codes
296	* 7822	**Mass, lump, or localized swelling** in abdomen, pelvis, chest, head & neck, skin & subcutaneous tissues *excl.* breast (611-), swelling of joint (7190), enlarged lymph node (7856)	L	782.2, 784.2, 786.6, 789.3
-		**Headache NOS (7840)**		
297	* 797-	**Senility, senescence** *excl.* senile dementia (294-)		797
-		**Behaviour disorder (312-)**		

Investigations with unexplained abnormal results
Urinanalysis

-		**Hematuria NOS (5997)**		
-		**Bacteriuria (595-)**		
298	* 791-	**Other abnormal urine test finding** *incl.* proteinuria *excl.* orthostatic albuminuria (5936), metabolic disorders involving amino acids & certain carbohydrates (279-)	M	791

Hematology

-		**Abnormal white cells** (in quality or quantity) **(288-)**		
-		**Abnormal platelets & coagulation tests (287-)**		
(375)	* 7900	**Other hematological abnormality** *incl.* red cells, raised ESR *excl.* anemia (280-, 281-, 282-, 285-, 648-), polycythemia rubra vera (239-)	N	790.0, 790.1

Position no.	ICHPPC code	List of diseases, disorders, and health problems	Changes from ICHPPC-1	Comparable ICD-9 codes

Blood chemistry

(51)   *** 7902**   **Abnormal unexplained biochemical test** *incl.* glucose tolerance test, multiphasic biochemical screening (SMA), bacteremia *excl.* disorders of: fluids, electrolytes, acid–base balance (279-), aminoacids & certain carbohydrates (279-), lipids (272-), renal failure, uremia (598-), hyperuricemia (274-), hypoglycemia (279-), hyperglycemia (250-)   L   790.2–790.9

(376)   *** 7950**   **Non-specific abnormal pap smear** *excl.* cervical dysplasia (622-), carcinoma-*in-situ* of cervix (180-)   N   795.0

(119)   *** 7962**   **Elevated blood-pressure without a diagnosis of hypertension** (hyperpiesia, hyperpiesis)   796.2

299   *** 793-**   **Other investigations with unexplained abnormal results** *incl.* ECG, X-rays, ultrasound, function studies, serology, histology   M   792–794, 795 ex. 795.0, 796 ex. 796.2

All other signs, symptoms, & ill-defined conditions

300   **7889**   **All other signs, symptoms, & ill-defined conditions** *incl.* abnormal gait, ataxia, jaundice, cyanosis, pallor, halitosis, gangrene, hiccough, fecal incontinence, ascites, death of unknown or undetermined cause, respiratory failure, other poorly understood condition which is under observation *excl.* stridor (7860), fluid & electrolyte disturbance (279-)   L   780.0, 780.1, 780.5, 780.9, 781 ex. 781.0, 782.4–782.9, 783.1, 783.5–783.9, 784.1, 784.6, 784.8, 784.9, 785.0, 785.3–785.5, pt. 785.9, 786.4, 786.7–786.9, 787.2, 787.4–787.9, 788.0, 788.2, 788.5–788.9, 789.4–789.9, 798, 799 (ex. 799.3, 799.4)

Position no.	ICHPPC code	List of diseases, disorders, and health problems	Changes from ICHPPC-1	Comparable ICD-9 codes

XVII. ACCIDENTS, INJURY, POiSONING, & VIOLENCE

Fractures (excl. malunion, non-union (739-))

301	802-	Skull & facial bones		800–804
302	805-	Vertebral column, with or without cord lesion		805, 806
303	807-	Ribs		807.0, 807.1
304	810-	Clavicle		810
305	812-	Humerus		812
306	813-	Radius, ulna *incl.* Colles' fracture		813
307	814-	Carpal, metacarpal, tarsal, metatarsal bone(s)		814, 815, 825
308	816-	Phalanges of foot or hand		816, 826
309	820-	Femur		820, 821
310	823-	Tibia, fibula *incl.* Pott's fracture		823, 824
311	829-	All other specified, or ill-defined fractures		807.2–807.6, 808, 809, 811, 817–819, 822, 827–829

Dislocations

312	836-	Acute damage to meniscus of knee *excl.* chronic damage to meniscus (717-)	L	836.0–836.2
313	839-	All other dislocations & subluxations	L	830–835, 836.3 –836.6, 837–839

Position no	ICHPPC code	List of diseases, disorders, and health problems	Changes from ICHPPC-1	Comparable ICD-9 codes

Sprains & strains (of joints, muscles, & ligaments)

314	840-	Shoulder, upper arm, elbow, forearm	W	840, 841
315	842-	Wrist, hand, finger		842
316	844-	Knee, (lower) leg		844
317	8450	Ankle		845.0
318	8451	Foot, toe		845.1
319	8470	Neck *incl.* whiplash		847.0
320	8478	Rest of vertebral column *incl.* sacroiliac region, coccyx		846, 847.1–847.9
321	848-	All other sprains & strains *incl.* ill-defined		843, 848

Other trauma

322	850-	Head injury, concussion, intracranial injury; without skull fracture *excl.* late effects (908), psychological effects (316-)		850–854
323	889-	Laceration, open wound, traumatic amputation *incl.* injuries to teeth & eardrum, puncture wound & animal bite	M	870–897
325	910-	Insect bite & sting		pt. 910–919, pt. 989.5
326	918-	Abrasion, scratch, blister *incl.* eye abrasion		pt. 910–919
327	929-	Bruise, contusion, crushing with intact skin surface *incl.* hematoma, contusion of eye *excl.* spontaneous subconjunctival hemorrhage (378-), internal organ injury (959-)		920–929
328	949-	Burns, scalds—all degrees *incl.* chemical burns, radiation burns, burns of eye		940–949

Position no.	ICHPPC code	List of diseases, disorders, and health problems	Changes from ICHPPC-1	Comparable ICD-9 codes
329	* 912-	**Foreign body in superficial tissues** *excl.* foreign body in eye (930-), residual or old foreign body in tissues, foreign body granuloma (728-)	W	pt. 910–919
330	930-	**Foreign body in eye** *incl.* adnexae *excl.* residual or old foreign body in eye (378-)	W	930
331	939-	**Foreign body entering through orifice** *excl.* eye		931–939
332	* 908-	**Late effects of trauma** *incl.* scarring, deformities, disabilities *excl.* non-union, malunion of fracture (739-)		905–909
333	959-	**Other injury or trauma** *incl.* multiple trauma, internal injury of chest, abdomen, and pelvis, laceration and other injury to nerve, early complications of trauma NOTE: for *suicide* or *attempted suicide*, code the nature of the self-inflicted injury or adverse effect as well as the any known underlying emotional or social problem	W	860–869, 900–904, 950–959

Adverse effects

Position no.	ICHPPC code	List of diseases, disorders, and health problems	Changes from ICHPPC-1	Comparable ICD-9 codes
334	977-	**Poisoning by medicinal agent, accidental or deliberate overdose**	M	960–979
(377)	* 9952	**Adverse effect of medicinal agent correctly administered in proper dosage** May also code the nature of the adverse effect *excl.* reaction to immunization & transfusion—(998-)	N	995.2
335	989-	**Toxic effects of other substances** *incl.* lead, carbon monoxide, industrial materials, poisonous plants	W	980–989 ex. pt. 989.5

Position no.	ICHPPC code	List of diseases, disorders, and health problems	Changes from ICHPPC-1	Comparable ICD-9 codes
336	998-	**Complications of surgery & medical treatment** *incl.* post-operative wound infection, hemorrhage, and disruption; complications of prostheses, devices, and implants; immunization & transfusion reactions *excl.* adverse effects of diagnostic & therapeutic X-rays (994-)	M	996–999
337	994-	**Adverse effects of physical factors** *incl.* heat, cold (incl. chilblains), pressure, motion, lightning, drowning, radiation (natural, industrial, diagnostic or therapeutic) *excl.* sunburn (692-), snowblindness (378-), radiation-burn (949-)	M	990–994
(378)	* 9950	**Certain adverse effects not elsewhere classified** *incl.* anaphylactic shock, angioneurotic edema, allergic edema, allergic reaction NOS, anesthetic shock	N	995 ex. 995.2

Position no.	ICHPPC code	List of diseases, disorders, and health problems	Changes from ICHPPC-1	Comparable ICD-9 codes

XVIII. SUPPLEMENTARY CLASSIFICATION

Preventive medicine

338	* V70-	**Medical examination** (where this is considered to be a reason for the contact), *incl.* health screening, complete or partial check-ups, care of well child or infant, pre-operative examination, cytology smear, examination or investigation to exclude specific disease	M	V20, V21, V28, V30–V39, V65.2, V65.5, V70, V71, V72 ex. V72.7, V73–V82
339	* V01-	**Contacts & carriers (suspected or proven) of infective or parasitic diseases** *incl.* prophylactic therapy *excl.* rheumatic fever prophylaxis (390-)		V01, V02, V07 ex. V07.
		Positive skin test conversion for tuberculosis (011-)		
		Allergy tests (code the allergy)		
340	* V03-	**Prophylactic immunization, innoculation, & vaccination**		V03–V06
341	* V14-	**Observation & care of patient on high risk medication** Requires: additional code for primary diagnosis		No equivalent *ICD-9* code
342	* V10-	**Observation & care of other high-risk patients** *incl.* patient-care management of prosthetic devices & implants, status post-surgery, family history of certain diseases, personal history of certain diseases	W	V10–V13, V15–V19, V42–V46 (ex. V45.5)

Family planning

343	* V252	**Sterilization of male or female**		pt. V25.0, pt. V25.4

Position no.	ICHPPC code	List of diseases, disorders, and health problems	Changes from ICHPPC-1	Comparable ICD-9 codes
344	* V255	Oral contraceptive		pt. V25.0, pt. V25.4
-		Complication of oral contraceptive (9952)		
345	* V251	Intrauterine device		V25.1, pt. V25.4, V45.5
346	* V253	Other method of contraception		V25.3, pt. V25.4, V25.8, V25.9
-		Complication of contraceptive device (998-)		
347	* V256	General contraceptive advice *incl.* advice about sterilization or therapeutic abortion	W	pt. V25.0

Administrative procedures

348	* V680	Letters, forms, certificates, and prescriptions without need for additional examination or interview of patient *excl.* prescription for oral contraceptive (V255)		V68 (ex. pt. V68.8)
349	* V683	Referral of patient without need for examination or interview		pt. V68.8

Maternal & child health care

350	* V223	The diagnosis of pregnancy		pt. V22.0–V22.2
351	* V220	Prenatal care, incidentally noted to be pregnant	W	pt. V22.0–V22.2, V23
		Requires: additional code for: complication of pregnancy (640- to 648-), associated non-obstetrical condition (passim)		
352	* V24-	Postpartum care (of mother) *excl.* suppression of lactation (676-)	L	V24
-		Well baby care (V70-)		

Position no.	ICHPPC code	List of diseases, disorders, and health problems	Changes from ICHPPC-1	Comparable ICD-9 codes

Miscellaneous

353	* V50-	**Medical or surgical procedure without reported diagnosis** *incl.* surgical assist, piercing of ears, circumcision without disease		V50, V51
354	* V654	**Advice, health instruction & education** *incl.* class instruction *excl.* contraceptive instruction (V256)	W	V26.3, V26.4, V65.3, V65.4
355	* V651	**Problems external to patient** *incl.* manifestation of anxiety in a third party, consulting for another (e.g. sick relative), blood donor	W	V59, V65.1

Social, marital, & family problems and maladjustments

Note: this section is for social problems and maladjustments (inside the family or outside) which have been explicitly discussed and which are accepted by the patient as a significant problem. More than one of these codes may be applied to a patient. These codes may be used alone to describe the substance of an encounter, or may be used as additional codes to show the interdependence between organic or mental disease and the social milieu of the patient *excl.* contact with person acting as emissary for another person who is experiencing problems (V651)

356	* V602	**Economic problem, poverty**	W	V60.2
357	* V600	**Housing problem**		V60.0, V60.1
358	* V614	**Problem of caring for sick person** (e.g. alcoholic family member) *excl.* patient lacking person able to render care (V624)	M	V61.4
359	* V611	**Marital problem** *incl.* problems of the relationship between a man & a woman, whether married or not *excl.* problems limited to sexual activity (3027)	M	V61.1
360	* V612	**Parent–child problem** *incl.* concern about behaviour of child, problems related to adopted or foster child, child abuse, battered child, child neglect		V61.2

Position no.	ICHPPC code	List of diseases, disorders, and health problems	Changes from ICHPPC-1	Comparable ICD-9 codes
361	* **V613**	**Problem with aged parents or in-laws**		V61.3
362	* **V610**	**Family disruption,** with or without divorce, affecting the couple or others *excl.* bereavement (308-)		V61.0
363	* **V619**	**Other problem of the family relationship NEC**		V61.5, V61.7–V61.9
364	* **V623**	**Educational problem**		V62.3
365	* **V616**	**Pregnancy out of wedlock (illegitimate pregnancy), illegitimacy**	W	V61.6
366	* **V624**	**Social maladjustment** *incl.* social isolation, persecution, cultural deprivation, political, religious, or sex discrimination	L	V62.4, V60.3–V60.6
367	* **V620**	**Occupational problem** *incl.* unemployment, difficulties at work or in adjusting to work situation, career choice problem or frustration		V62.0–V62.2
368	* **V627**	**Phase-of-life social problem NEC**	L	pt. V62.8
(370)	* **V625**	**Legal problem** *incl.* imprisonment, prosecution, litigation, legal investigations		V62.5
369	* **V629**	**Other social problems** *incl.* refusal of treatment for reasons of religion or conscience	W	V60.8, V60.9, V62.6–V62.9 (ex. pt. V62.8)

Other problems not classifiable elsewhere

371	* **V999**	**All other problems not classifiable in codes 008- to V629** *incl.* disfigurement or cosmetic problem NOS, other supplementary classification options detailed in ICD.	L	V07.1, V14, V25.4, V26 (ex. V26.3, V26.4), V27, V40, V41, V47–V49, V52–V58, V63, V64, V65.0, V65.8, V65.9, V66, V67, V72.7

Appendix: Condensed titles for machine processing and computer printouts

This list of condensed diagnostic titles is designed for machine processing and computer printouts. Each title contains a maximum of 35 letters and spaces. It is necessary to refer to the tabular section for the full content of each rubric. The following abbreviations and symbols are used:

&	and, and/or
/	and/or
EXCL	excluding
INCL	including
NEC	not elsewhere classified
NOS	not otherwise specified
NYD	not yet diagnosed
WO	without
W/WO	with or without

Position no.	ICHPPC code	Condensed title

I. INFECTIVE & PARASITIC DISEASES

1	008-	PROVEN INFECTIOUS INTESTINE DISEASE
2	009-	PRESUMED INFECTIOUS INTESTIN DISEAS
4	011-	TUBERCULOSIS
6	033-	WHOOPING COUGH
7	034-	STREP THROAT, SCARLET FEV, ERYSIPELAS
8	045-	POLIO & CNS ENTEROVIRAL DISEASES
9	052-	CHICKENPOX
10	053-	HERPES ZOSTER
11	054-	HERPES SIMPLEX
12	055-	MEASLES
13	056-	RUBELLA
14	057-	OTHER VIRAL EXANTHEMS
15	070-	INFECTIOUS HEPATITIS
16	072-	MUMPS
17	075-	INFECTIOUS MONONUCLEOSIS
18	077-	VIRAL CONJUNCTIVITIS
19	0781	WARTS, ALL SITES
20	0799	VIRAL INFECTION NOS
21	084-	MALARIA
22	090-	SYPHILIS, ALL SITES & STAGES
23	098-	GONORREA, ALL SITES
372	0994	NON-SPECIFIC URETHRITIS
24	110-	DERMATOPHYTOSIS & DERMATOMYCOSIS
25	112-	MONILIASIS EXCL UROGENITAL
26	1121	MONILIASIS, UROGENITAL, PROVEN
27	1310	TRICHOMONIASIS, UROGENITAL, PROVEN
28	127-	OXYURIASIS, PINWORMS, HELMINTH NEC
29	132-	PEDICULOSIS & OTHER INFESTATIONS
30	133-	SCABIES & OTHER ACARIASIS
31	136-	OTHER INFECT/PARASITIC DISEASES NEC

Position no.	ICHPPC code	Condensed title

II. NEOPLASMS

Malignant neoplasms

32	151-	MALIG NEOPL GASTROINTESTINAL TRACT
33	162-	MALIGNANT NEOPL RESPIRATORY TRACT
34	173-	MALIG NEOPL SKIN/SUBCUTANEOUS TISSU
35	174-	MALIGNANT NEOPLASM BREAST
36	180-	MALIG NEOPL FEMALE GENITAL TRACT
37	188-	MALIG NEOPL URINARY & MALE GENITAL
38	201-	HODGKINS DISEASE, LYMPHOMA, LEUKEMIA
39	199-	OTHER MALIGNANT NEOPLASMS NEC

Benign neoplasms

40	214-	LIPOMA, ANY SITE
41	216-	BENIGN NEOPLASM SKIN
42	217-	BENIGN NEOPLASM BREAST
43	218-	BENIGN NEOPLASM UTERUS
44	228-	HEMANGIOMA & LYMPHANGIOMA
45	229-	OTHER BENIGN NEOPLASMS NEC

Unspecified neoplasms

46	239-	NEOPL NYD AS BENIGN OR MALIGNANT

Position no.	ICHPPC code	Condensed title

III. ENDOCR, NUTRIT, METABOL DISEAS

47	240-	NONTOXIC GOITER & NODULE
48	242-	THYROTOXICOSIS W/WO GOITER
49	244-	HYPOTHYROIDISM, MYXEDEMA, CRETINISM
50	250-	DIABETES MELLITUS
52	260-	AVITAMIN & NUTRITIONAL DISORDER NEC
54	274-	GOUT
55	278-	OBESITY
56	272-	LIPID METABOLISM DISORDERS
57	279-	OTHER ENDOCR, NUTRITN, METABOL DISORD

Position no.	ICHPPC code	Condensed title

IV. BLOOD DISEASES

58	280-	IRON DEFICIENCY ANEMIA
59	281-	PERNICIOUS & OTHER DEFICIENC ANEMIA
60	282-	HEREDITARY HEMOLYTIC ANEMIAS
61	285-	ANEMIA, OTHER/UNSPECIFIED
62	287-	PURPURA, HEMORRHAG & COAGULAT DEFECT
63	2891	LYMPHADENITIS, CHRONIC/NONSPECIFIC
64	288-	ABNORMAL WHITE CELLS
65	2899	BLOOD/BLOOD FORMING ORGAN DISOR NEC

Position no.	ICHPPC code	Condensed title

V. MENTAL DISORDERS

Psychoses except alcoholic

66	294-	ORGANIC PSYCHOSIS EXCL ALCOHOLIC
67	295-	SCHIZOPHRENIA, ALL TYPES
68	296-	AFFECTIVE PSYCHOSES
69	298-	PSYCHOSIS, OTHER/NOS EXCL ALCOHOLIC

Neuroses

70	3000	ANXIETY DISORDER
71	3001	HYSTERICAL & HYPOCHONDRIAC DISORDER
72	3004	DEPRESSIVE DISORDER
73	3009	NEUROSIS, OTHER/UNSPECIFIED

Other mental, psycholog disorders

74	315-	SPECIFIC LEARNING DISTURBANCE
75	3074	INSOMNIA & OTHER SLEEP DISORDERS
76	3078	TENSION HEADACHE
77	308-	TRANSIEN SITUAT DISTURB, ADJ REACT
78	312-	BEHAVIOR DISORDERS NEC
79	3027	SEXUAL PROBLEMS
80	3031	ALCOHOL ABUSE & ALCOHOLIC PSYCHOSIS
81	3050	ACUTE ALCOHOLIC INTOXICATION
82	3051	TOBACCO ABUSE
83	3048	OTHER DRUG ABUSE, HABIT, ADDICTION
84	301-	PERSONALITY & CHARACTER DISORDERS
85	317-	MENTAL RETARDATION
86	316-	OTHER MENTAL & PSYCHOLOGIC DISORDER

Position no.	ICHPPC code	Condensed title

VI. NERV SYSTEM, SENSE ORGAN DISEAS

Nervous system diseases

87	340-	MULTIPLE SCLEROSIS
88	332-	PARKINSONISM
89	345-	EPILEPSY, ALL TYPES
90	346-	MIGRAINE
91	355-	OTHER NERVOUS SYSTEM DISEASES NEC

Eye diseases

92	3720	CONJUNCTIVITIS & OPHTHALMIA
93	3730	EYELID INFECTIONS/CHALAZION
94	367-	REFRACTIVE ERRORS
96	366-	CATARACT
97	365-	GLAUCOMA
98	369-	BLINDNESS
99	378-	OTHER EYE DISEASES

Ear diseases

100	3801	OTITIS EXTERNA
101	3820	ACUTE OTITIS MEDIA
102	3811	ACUTE & CHRON SEROUS OTITIS MED
103	3815	EUSTACHIAN BLOCK OR CATARRH
104	386-	VERTIGINOUS SYNDROMES
105	387-	DEAFNESS, PARTIAL OR COMPLETE
106	3804	WAX IN EAR
107	388-	OTHER EAR & MASTOID DISEASES

Position no.	ICHPPC code	Condensed title

VII. CIRCULATORY SYSTEM DISEASES

Heart diseases

108	390-	RHEUMATIC FEVER/HEART DISEASE
109	410-	AC MYOCARD INFARCT/SUBAC ISCHEMIA
110	412-	CHRONIC ISCHEMIC HEART DISEASE
112	428-	HEART FAILURE, RIGHT/LEFT SIDED
113	4273	ATRIAL FIBRILLATION OF FLUTTER
114	4270	PAROXYSMAL TACHYCARDIA
115	4276	ECTOPIC BEATS, ALL TYPES
117	416-	PULMONARY HEART DISEASE
111	424-	DISEAS HEART VALV NON-RHEUM, NOS, NYD
118	429-	OTHER HEART DISEASES NEC

Blood pressure problems

120	401-	HYPERTENSION, UNCOMPLICATED
121	402-	HYPERTENSION INVOLVING TARGET ORGAN

Vascular system diseases

123	435-	TRANSIENT CEREBRAL ISCHEMIA
124	438-	OTHER CEREBROVASCULAR DISEASE
125	440-	ATHEROSCLEROSIS EXCL HEART & BRAIN
126	443-	OTHER ARTERIAL DISEAS EXCL ANEURYSM
127	415-	PULMONARY EMBOLISM & INFARCTION
128	451-	PHLEBITIS & THROMBOPHLEBITIS
129	454-	VARICOSE VEINS OF LEGS
130	455-	HEMORRHOIDS
131	4580	POSTURAL HYPOTENSION
132	459-	OTHER PERIPHERAL VESSEL DISEASES

Position no.	ICHPPC code	Condensed title

VIII. RESPIRATORY SYSTEM DISEASES

133	460-	ACUTE UPPER RESPIR TRACT INFECTION
134	461-	SINUSITIS, ACUTE & CHRONIC
135	463-	ACUTE TONSILLITIS & QUINSY
136	474-	HYPERTROPH/CHRON INFECT TONSL/ADEN
137	464-	LARYNGITIS & TRACHEITIS, ACUTE
138	466-	BRONCHITIS, & BRONCHIOLITIS, ACUTE
139	487-	INFLUENZA
140	486-	PNEUMONIA
141	5110	PLEURISY ALL TYPES EXCL TUBERCUL
5	5119	PLEURAL EFFUSION NOS
142	491-	BRONCHITIS, CHRONIC & BRONCHIECTASIS
143	492-	EMPHYSEMA & COPD
144	493-	ASTHMA
145	477-	HAY FEVER
146	4781	BOIL IN NOSE
147	519-	OTHER RESPIRATORY SYSTEM DISEASES

Position no.	ICHPPC code	Condensed title

X. GENITOURINARY SYSTEM DISEASES

Urinary system diseases

168	580-	GLOMERULONEPHRITIS, ACUTE & CHRONIC
169	5901	PYELONEPHRITIS & PYELITIS, ACUTE
170	595-	CYSTITIS & URINARY INFECTION NOS
171	592-	URINARY SYSTEM CALCULUS, ALL TYPES
172	597-	URETHRITIS NOS, NEC
173	5936	ORTHOSTATIC ALBUMINURIA
373	5997	HEMATURIA NOS
174	598-	OTHER URINARY SYSTEM DISEASES NEC

Male genital organ diseases

175	600-	BENIGN PROSTATIC HYPERTROPHY
176	601-	PROSTATIS & SEMINAL VESICULITIS
177	603-	HYDROCELE
178	604-	ORCHITIS & EPIDIDYMITIS
179	605-	REDUND PREPUCE, PHIMOSIS & BALANITIS
180	607-	OTHER MALE GENITAL ORGAN DISEASES

Breast diseases

181	610-	CHRONIC CYSTIC BREAST DISEASE
182	611-	OTHER BREAST DISEASES

Female genital organ diseases

183	614-	PELVIC INFLAMMATORY DISEASE
184	622-	CERVICITIS & CERVICAL EROSION
185	6161	VAGINITIS NOS, VULVITIS
186	618-	UTEROVAGINAL PROLAPSE
187	627-	MENOPAUSAL SYMPTOMS & POST MENO BLEED
188	6254	PREMENSTRUAL TENSION SYNDROME
374	6250	NON-PSYCH VAGINISMUS & DYSPAREUNIA

Position no.	ICHPPC code	Condensed title

Disorders of menstruation

189	6260	ABSENT, SCANTY, RARE MENSTRUATION
190	6262	EXCESSIVE MENSTRUATION
191	6253	PAINFUL MENSTRUATION
193	6269	INTERMENSTR BLEEDING
194	629-	OTHER FEMALE GENITAL ORGAN DISEASES

Fertility problems

195	606-	STERILITY & REDUCED FERTILITY

Position no.	ICHPPC code	Condensed title

XI. PREGNANCY, CHILDBIRTH, PUERPERIUM

196	633-	ECTOPIC PREGNANCY
197	640-	BLEEDING DURING PREGNANY
198	6466	URINARY INFECTION, PREG & POSTPART
199	642-	TOXEMIAS OF PREG & PUERPERIUM
200	636-	INDUCED ABORTION
201	634-	ABORTION, SPONTANEOUS & NOS
202	648-	OTHER COMPLICATIONS OF PREGNANCY
203	650-	NORMAL DELIVERY
204	661-	COMPLICATED DELIVERY
205	676-	MASTITIS & LACTATION DISORDERS
206	670-	OTHER COMPLICATIONS OF PUERPERIUM

Position no.	ICHPPC code	Condensed title

XII. SKIN, SUBCUTANEOUS TISSU DISEAS

207	680-	BOIL & CELLULITIS INCL FINGR & TOE
209	683-	LYMPHADENITIS, ACUTE
210	684-	IMPETIGO
211	685-	OTHER INFECTIONS SKIN/SUBCUTANEOUS
212	690-	SEBORRHOEIC DERMATITIS
213	6918	ECZEMA & ALLERGIC DERMATITIS
214	692-	CONTACT & OTHER DERMATITIS NEC
215	6910	DIAPER RASH
216	6963	PITYRIASIS ROSEA
217	6961	PSORIASIS W/WO ARTHROPATHY
218	698-	PRURITIS & RELATED CONDITIONS
219	700-	CORNS & CALLOSITIES
220	7062	SEBACEOUS CYST
221	703-	INGROWN TOENAIL & NAIL DISEASE NEC
222	704-	ALOPECIA & OTHER HAIR DISEASES
223	705-	POMPHOLYX & SWEAT GLAND DIS NEC
224	7061	ACNE
225	707-	CHRONIC SKIN ULCER
226	708-	URTICARIA
227	709-	OTHER SKIN & SUBCUTANE TISSU DISEAS

Position no.	ICHPPC code	Condensed title

XIII. MUSCULOSKELET, CONNECTIV TISSU DISEASE

Arthritis & arthrosis

228	714-	RHEUMATOID ARTHRIT & ALLIED CONDITN
229	715-	OSTEOARTHRITIS & ALLIED CONDITIONS
230	7161	TRAUMATIC ARTHRITIS
288	7194	PAIN OR STIFFNESS IN JOINT
289	7190	SWELLING OR EFFUSION OF JOINT
231	725-	ARTHRITIS NEC/DIFF CONN TISS DIS

Nonarticular rheumatism

232	7260	SHOULDER SYNDROMES
233	7263	OTHER BURSITIS & SYNOVITIS
234	728-	OTHER NONARTICULAR RHEUMATISM
286	7295	PAIN & OTHER LIMB SYMPTOMS

Vertebral column syndromes

235	723-	CERVICAL SPINE SYNDROMES
237	721-	OSTEOARTHRITIS OF SPINE
238	7242	BACK PAIN WO RADIATING SYMPTOMS
239	7244	BACK PAIN WITH RADIATING SYMPTOMS
240	737-	ACQUIRED DEFORMITIES OF SPINE

Other musculoskel, connect tiss disord

241	7274	GANGLION OF JOINT & TENDON
242	732-	OSTEOCHONDROSIS
243	7330	OSTEOPOROSIS
244	717-	CHRONIC INTERNAL KNEE DERANGEMENT
245	736-	ACQUIRED DEFORMITY OF LIMBS
246	739-	OTHER MUSCULOSKEL, CONNECTIV DISEAS

Position no.	ICHPPC code	Condensed title

XIV. CONGENITAL ANOMALIES

247	746-	CONGENITAL ANOMALY HEART & CIRCULAT
248	754-	CONGENITAL ANOMALIES OF LOWER LIMB
249	7525	UNDESCENDED TESTICLE
251	7436	BLOCKED TEAR DUCT
252	758-	OTHER CONGENITAL ANOMALIES NEC

Position	ICHPPC	
no.	code	Condensed title

XV. PERINATAL MORBIDITY & MORTALITY

| 253 | 778- | ALL PERINATAL CONDITIONS |

Position no.	ICHPPC code	Condensed title

XVI. SIGN, SYMPTOM, ILL DEFINED COND

Central & peripheral nerv system

254	7803	CONVULSIONS
255	7810	ABNORMAL INVOLUNTARY MOVEMENT
256	7804	DIZZINESS & GIDDINESS
257	7845	DISTURBANCE OF SPEECH
258	7840	HEADACHE
259	7820	DISTURBANCE OF SENSATION

Cardiovascular & lymphatic system

262	7865	CHEST PAIN
263	7851	PALPITATIONS
264	7802	SYNCOPE, FAINT, BLACKOUT
116	7852	HEART MURMUR NEC, NYD
265	7823	EDEMA
266	7856	ENLARGED LYMPH NODES, NOT INFECTED

Respiratory system

267	7847	EPISTAXIS
268	7863	HEMOPTYSIS
269	7860	DYSPNEA
270	7862	COUGH

Gastrointestinal system & abdomen

273	7830	ANOREXIA
274	7870	NAUSEA/VOMITING
275	7871	HEARTBURN
277	7891	HEPATOMEGALY/SPLENOMEGALY
278	7873	FLATULENCE, BLOATING, ERUCTATION
279	7890	ABDOMINAL PAIN

Position no.	ICHPPC code	Condensed title

Genitourinary system

280	7881	DYSURIA
281	7883	ENURESIS
283	7884	FREQUENCY OF URINATION

General signs & symptoms

290	7808	EXCESSIVE SWEATING
291	7806	FEVER OF UNDETERMINED CAUSE
292	7821	RASH & OTHER NONSPECIFIC SKIN ERUPT
293	7832	WEIGHT LOSS
294	7834	LACK OF EXPECTED PHYSIOLOG DEVELOP
53	7833	FEEDING PROBLEM BABY OR ELDERLY
295	7807	MALAISE, FATIGUE, TIREDNESS
296	7822	MASS & LOCALIZED SWELLING NOS/NYD
297	797-	SENILITY WITHOUT PSYCHOSIS

Unexplained abnormal results

Urinanalysis

298	791-	ABNORMAL URINE TEST NEC

Hematology

375	7900	HEMATOLOGICAL ABNORMALITY NEC

Blood chemistry

51	7902	ABNORMAL UNEXPLAINED BIOCHEM TEST

Other abnormal results

376	7950	NON-SPECIFIC ABNORMAL PAP SMEAR
119	7962	ELEVATED BLOOD PRESSURE
299	793-	OTHER UNEXPLAINED ABNORMAL RESULTS

Position no.	ICHPPC code	Condensed title

Sign, symptom, ill defined cond NEC

| *300* | 7889 | SIGN, SYMPTOM, ILL DEFINED COND NEC |

Position no.	ICHPPC code	Condensed title

XVII. INJURIES & ADVERSE EFFECTS

Fractures

301	802-	FRACTURE SKULL & FACIAL BONES
302	805-	FRACTURE VERTEBRAL COLUMN
303	807-	FRACTURE RIBS
304	810-	FRACTURE CLAVICLE
305	812-	FRACTURE HUMERUS
306	813-	FRACTURE RADIUS/ULNA
307	814-	FRACT (META)CARPAL & (META)TARSAL
308	816-	FRACTURE PHALANGES FOOT/HAND
309	820-	FRACTURE FEMUR
310	823-	FRACTURE TIBIA/FIBULA
311	829-	FRACTURE ALL OTHER SITES NEC

Dislocations & subluxations

312	836-	ACUTE DAMAGE KNEE MENISCUS
313	839-	DISLOC/SUBLUX OTHER SITES NEC

Sprains & strains

314	840-	SPRAIN/STRAIN SHOULDER & ARM
315	842-	SPRAIN/STRAIN WRIST, HAND, FINGERS
316	844-	SPRAIN/STRAIN KNEE & LOWER LEG
317	8450	SPRAIN/STRAIN ANKLE
318	8451	SPRAIN/STRAIN FOOT & TOES
319	8470	SPRAIN/STRAIN NECK
320	8478	SPRAIN/STRAIN VERTEBRAL EXCL NECK
321	848-	SPRAIN & STRAIN ALL OTHER SITES NEC

Position no.	ICHPPC code	Condensed title

Other traumas

322	850-	CONCUSSION & INTRACRANIAL INJURY
823	889-	LACERAT/OPEN WOUND/TRAUM AMPUTATN
325	910-	INSECT BITES & STINGS
326	918-	ABRASION, SCRATCH, BLISTER
327	929-	BRUISE, CONTUSION, CRUSHING
328	949-	BURNS & SCALDS, ALL DEGREES
329	912-	FOREIGN BODY IN TISSUES
330	930-	FOREIGN BODY IN EYE
331	939-	FOREIGN BODY ENTERING THRU ORIFICE
332	908-	LATE EFFECT OF TRAUMA
333	959-	OTHER INJURIES & TRAUMA

Adverse effects

334	977-	OVERDOS MEDICIN ACCID OR DELIBERAT
377	9952	ADVERS EFFECT MEDICIN PROPER DOSE
335	989-	ADVERSE EFFECTS OF OTHER CHEMICALS
336	998-	SURGERY & MEDICAL CARE COMPLICATION
337	994-	ADVERSE EFFECTS OF PHYSICAL FACTORS
378	9950	OTHER ADVERSE EFFECTS NEC

Position no.	ICHPPC code	Condensed title

SUPPLEMENTARY CLASSIFICATION

Preventive medicine

338	V70-	MEDICAL EXAM
339	V01-	CONTAC/CARRIER, INFEC/PARASIT DIS
340	V03-	PROPHYLACTIC IMMUNIZATION
341	V14-	OBSERV/CARE PT ON HI RISK MEDICAT
342	V10-	OBSERV/CARE OTHER HI RISK PATIENT

Family planning

343	V252	STERILIZATION OF MALE OR FEMALE
344	V255	ORAL CONTRACEPTIVES
345	V251	INTRAUTERINE DEVICES
346	V253	OTHER CONTRACEPTIVE METHODS
347	V256	GENERAL CONTRACEPTIVE GUIDANCE

Administrative procedures

348	V680	LETTER, FORMS, PRESCRIPTION WO EXAM
349	V683	REFERRAL WO EXAM OR INTERVIEW

Maternal & child health care

350	V223	DIAGNOSING PREGNANCY
351	V220	PRENATAL CARE
352	V24-	POSTNATAL CARE

Miscellaneous

353	V50-	MED/SURG PROCEDURE WO DIAGNOSIS
354	V654	ADVICE & HEALTH INSTRUCTION
355	V651	PROBLEMS EXTERNAL TO PATIENT

Position no.	ICHPPC code	Condensed title

Social, marital, family problems

356	V602	ECONOMIC PROBLEM
357	V600	HOUSING PROBLEM
358	V614	MEDICAL CARE PROBLEM
359	V611	MARITAL PROBLEM
360	V612	PARENT & CHILD PROBLEM
361	V613	AGED PARENT OR INLAW PROBLEM
362	V610	FAMILY DISRUPTION W/WO DIVORCE
363	V619	OTHER FAMILY PROBLEMS
364	V623	EDUCATIONAL PROBLEM
365	V616	PREGNANCY OUT OF WEDLOCK
366	V624	SOCIAL MALADJUSTMENT
367	V620	OCCUPATIONAL PROBLEM
368	V627	PHASE-OF-LIFE PROBLEM NEC
370	V625	LEGAL PROBLEM
369	V629	OTHER SOCIAL PROBLEM

Other problems NEC

371	V999	PROBLEMS NEC IN CODES 008- TO V629

Alphabetical index

The ICHPPC alphabetical index does not contain all of the variations and synonyms of terms found in the tabular section which should be consulted as the primary coding instrument. It does, however, contain several diagnostic titles which are not found in the tabular section. For terms not listed in this index, the recorder is advised to consult volume 2, Alphabetical Index of the *International Classification of Diseases,* ninth Revision (*ICD–9*).

As with the index of ICD–9 this section is organized in the form of lead terms (main entries) at the left of the column, with various levels of indentation that identify the variations or anatomical sites. Usually the lead term is the name of the disease or health problem. For the supplementary section, chapter XVIII, key words such as 'counselling' and 'examination' are the main entries.

The code numbers found in the alphabetical index are those assigned to *ICHPPC–2.* Equivalent *ICD–9* code numbers and position numbers may be obtained by consulting the tabular section. Abbreviations are the same as those listed in the introduction. Parentheses are used to enclose synonyms or explanatory phrases that may or may not be present in the diagnostic title. Spelling is consistent with United States convention. Familiarity with the contents of the tabular section will make this alphabetical index more useful.

Abscess (*cont.*)
stitch 998-
subcutaneous 680-
thumb 680-
toe 680-
tonsil 463-
vagina 6161
vulva 629-
Absence (of)
acquired
  extremities, any part 736-
  eye 378-
  teeth, complete or partial 520-
congenital
  cardiovascular 746-
  chin 758-
  ear 758-
  lower limb(s) (hip) 754-
Absorption
disturbance of, fat or protein 578-
narcotic through placenta, fetus
      or newborn 778-
Abuse
alcohol 3050
  acute intoxication 3050
  chronic 3031
  nondependent 3050
alcoholism 3031
child V612
diazepam 3048
glue 3048
hallucinogen 3048
laxatives 3048
narcotic 3048
opiate 3048
psychostimulant 3048
tobacco smoking 3051
Acanthosis nigricans 709-
Acariasis 133-
Accessory, congenital
heart 746-
lower limb 758-
site, other NEC 758-
vascular 746-
Accident, cerebrovascular 438-
Acetonemia 7902
Acetonuria 791
Achalasia 530-
psychogenic 3001
Achlorhydria NOS 536-
anemia 280-
diarrhea 536-
neurogenic 536-

psychogenic 3001
secondary to vagotomy 579-
Acid intoxication 279-
Acidemia 279-
Acidity
gastric 536-
psychogenic 3001
Acidosis NOS 279-
diabetic 250-
metabolic NEC 279-
renal 598-
respiratory 279-
Acne 7061
Acrocyanosis 443-
Acrodermatitis (continua) 685-
Acromegaly 279-
Actinomycosis 136-
Addiction
alcohol 3031
drug (barbiturate) (hallucinogen) 3048
infant, chemical substance transmitted
      through placenta 778-
psychostimulant 3048
wine 3031
Addison's disease 279-
Adduction
foot 739-
  congenital 758-
hip 739-
  congenital 754-
Adenitis
acute NOS 683-
endemic infectious 075-
salivary glands 528-
Adenocarcinoma – *see* Neoplasm,
      malignant
Adenoiditis 474-
acute 463-
Adenoma
breast 217-
ovary 229-
prostate 600-
sebaceous 216-
site, other NEC—*see* 229-
thyroid 229-
  with hyperthyroidism or
        thyrotoxicosis 242-
uterus 218-
Adenomyosis 629-
Adenopathy 7856
Adenosis, breast 610-
Adhesions, adhesive
abdominal wall 579-

Adhesions, adhesive *(cont.)*
capsulitis, shoulder 7260
foreskin 605-
labium 758-
pelvic, female 614-
peritoneal 579-
pleura 5110
  tuberculous 011-
postpartal, old 629-
shoulder 726-
tongue 758-
Adiposity 278-
heart 429-
Adjustment reaction
adolescence 308-
adult or late life 308-
behavior disorder 312-
poor adjustment to illness V629
transient situational 308-
Adrenogenital syndrome 279-
Adynamic ileus 579-
Advice
family planning V256
health instruction or education V654
problems external to patient V651
Aerophagia 3001
Aftercare
checkup, no disease V70-
management of high-risk prosthetic
  device or implant V10-
patient on high-risk medication V14-
After-cataract 366-
Agalactia 676-
Agammaglobulinemia 279-
Agitation 316-
Agranulocytosis 288-
Albinism 279-
Albuminuria NOS 7900
arising during pregnancy 648-
orthostatic 5936
postural 5936
puerperal 648-
Alcoholism, alcoholic
acute intoxication 3031
addiction 3031
cardiopathy 3031
cirrhosis of liver 571-
delirium 3031
dementia 3031
gastritis, chronic 536-
hepatitis 571-
Aleukemia 201-
Alkalosis 279-

Allergy, allergic NOS 9950
due to
  adhesive tape 692-
  airborne substance 477-
  animal dander or hair 477-
  beesting (anaphylactic shock) 910-
  cold weather 692-
  cosmetic 692-
  detergent 692-
  drug (any) (external) (internal) 9952
    dermatitis 692-
    wrong substance or overdose 977-
  dust 477-
  dye 692-
  feathers 477-
  food 692-
    atopic 692-
  gastroenteritis or colitis 558-
  grass 477-
    asthmatic 493-
  heat or hot weather 692-
  inhalant 477-
  plant leaf contact 692-
  pollen (ragweed) 477-
    asthmatic 493-
  serum (anaphylactic shock) 998-
  solvent 692-
  tobacco 692-
Alopecia 704-
syphilitic 090-
Altitude, high, effect of 994-
Amaurosis fugax 378-
Amblyopia 378-
Ameba, amebic
carrier or suspected carrier V01-
coli 008-
Amebiasis, any site 008-
Amenorrhea 6260
Amino-acid deficiency 279-
Amnesia, hysterical or psychogenic 3001
Amputation
stump, painful or with
        late complications 998-
traumatic, any limb(s) 889-
Amputee 736-
Amyloidosis 279-
Anacidity, gastric 536-
psychogenic 3001
Anaphylactic shock or reaction 9950
following bite or sting 910-
from
  medicines 9950
  nonmedicinal agents 989-
  serum or immunization 998-

Anemia NOS 285-
achlorhydric 280-
agranulocytic 288-
aplastic 285-
atypical 285-
combined system disease 281-
Cooley's 282-
deficiency NOS 281-
  folic acid 281-
  iron 280-
  of pregnancy 648-
due to blood loss 280-
during pregnancy 648-
hemolytic NOS 282-
  acquired 285-
  hereditary 282-
hyperchromic 280-
  of pregnancy 648-
iron deficiency 280-
macrocytic 281-
  of pregnancy 648-
megaloblastic 281-
  of pregnancy 648-
  postpartum 648-
microcytic 280-
  familial 282-
myeloblastic or myelocytic 201-
newborn 778-
  posthemorrhagic 778-
normocytic NOS 285-
nutritional 281-
pernicious 281-
secondary 285-
sickle cell 282-
thrombocytopenic 287
Anesthesia
sensation 7820
surgical assist V50-
Aneurysm
abdominal 459-
aortic 459-
  valve 424-
carotid 459-
cerebrovascular (arteriosclerotic) 438-
congenital 746-
heart 412-
  acute 410-
site, other NEC 459-
valve 424-
Angiectasis 459-
Angiitis 459-
Angina (pectoris) 412-
Ludwig's 528-

Vincent's 136-
Angioedema 9950
Angiofibroma 229-
Angioma (benign) (cavernous) 228-
senile 459-
spider 459-
stellate 459-
Angiomatosis 758-
multiple sites 758-
Angioneurosis 3001
Angiospasm (traumatic) 443-
nerve 355-
Anisocoria 378-
Ankylosis, ankylosing
joint produced by surgical fusion V10-
sacroiliac 7242
spondylitis (spine) 714-
Anomaly
heart or circulatory structure 746-
lower limb 754-
site, other NEC 758-
toenail 758-
Anorexia NOS 7830
hysterical 3001
nervosa 316-
Anosmia 7889
hysterical 3001
Anovulatory cycle 606-
Anthracosilicosis 519-
Anxiety (neurosis) (reaction) (state) 3000
depression 3004
hysteria 3009
Aortic stenosis 424-
Aphakia, acquired 378-
Aphasia 7845
Apnea 7860
Appendicitis 540-
Appetite
depraved or perverted 316
excessive 7889
lack or loss of 7830
Arcus senilis 378-
Arrest, cardiac 429-
Arrhythmia NOS 429-
ectopic 4276
Arteriosclerosis or atherosclerosis
    (arteriosclerotic) NOS 440-
cardiovascular 412-
cerebral (brain) 438-
cerebrovascular 438-
extremities 440-
generalized 440-
heart disease NOS 412-

Attack (*cont.*)
rape 959-
  with injuries, code the injuries
syncope or faint 7802
vasovagal 7802
Avitamonosis 260-
Avulsion injury 889-
Awareness of heartbeat 7851
Ayerza's disease 416-
Azoospermia 606-
Azotemia 791-

Backache NOS 7242
postsurgical 739-
psychogenic 3078
Bacterial intestinal disease
presumed 009-
proven 008-
Bacteriuria, asymptomatic 595-
in pregnancy or puerperium 6466
Balanitis 605-
gonococcal 098-
Baldness 704-
Bamberger-Marie disease 739-
Barlow's disease 260-
Barrel chest 739-
Bartholin's
adenitis 629-
cyst 629-
gland abscess 629-
Basal cell cancer 199-
Battered baby or child V612
Beat—*see* Heartbeat
Bedsore 707-
Bedwetting 7883
Behavior—*see* Reaction
Belching 7873
Bicuspid aortic valve 746-
Bigeminy rhythm 429-
Biliary dyskinesia 574-
Birthmark, angiomatous 758-
Bites
animal 889-
chigger 133-
insect 910-
poisonous
  animal 989-
  insect 910-
reptile 989-
snake 989-
venomous—see Bites, poisonous
Black eye due to contusion 929-
Blackhead 7061

Blackout 7802
Blast injury—*see* 850 thru 959
Blastomycosis 136-
Bleeding—*see also* Hemorrhage
ear 388-
eye 378-
during pregnancy 640-
gastrointestinal NOS 578-
gums 520-
intermenstrual 6269
oral 528-
per rectum 5693
postmenopausal 627-
stools 578-
stump 998-
umbilical 778-
uterine 6269
vaginal 629-
Blennorrhea 098-
inclusion 778-
Blepharitis (bacterial) (seborrhoeic)
            (staphylococcal) (ulcerative) 3730
Blepharospasm 355-
Blindness
acquired or congenital one or both eyes 369-
color 378-
night 378-
word 315-
Blister, skin 918-
Bloating 7873
Block, blocked
eustachian tube 3815
heart (A-V) 429-
tear duct 378-
  congenital 7436
Blood donor V651
potential, examination of V70-
Bloody
discharge 7889
nose 7847
Bloodshot eyes 378-
Blue diaper syndrome 279-
Blurred vision 378-
Boil
auditory meatus, external 680-
axilla 680-
finger 680-
genital, male NEC 607-
groin 680-
nose
  inside 4781
  outside 680-
seminal vesicles 601-

Cellulitis (*cont.*)
male 607-
hand 680-
lips 528-
mouth 528-
nose, inside 519-
orbital 378-
perirectal 565-
site, other NEC 680-
thumb 680-
toe 680-
Cephalgia, nonorganic 3078
Cephalhematoma
birth injury 778-
other 929-
Cerebrovascular disease 438-
Certificate completion V680-
Cerumen 3804
Cervical
erosion 622-
rib syndrome 758-
root syndrome 723-
Cervicalgia 723-
Cervicitis 622-
Cervicobrachial syndrome 723-
Cestode infestation 127-
Chalazion 3730
Chancre 090-
Chancroid 136-
Change in bowel habits 579-
Chapping skin 709-
Charcot's joint 090-
nonvenereal 725-
Charley-horse, quadriceps 848-
Cheilitis 528-
Cheilosis angular 528-
Chemotherapy
maintenance V999
prophylactic NEC V01-
Chest-wall syndrome 7865
Chiari–Frommel syndrome 676-
Chickenpox 052-
Chigger bite 133-
Chilblains 994-
Chills 7889
Chloasma 709-
Choking 7889
Cholangitis 574-
Cholecystitis 574-
Cholecystolithiasis 574-
Choledocholithiasis 574-
Cholelithiasis 574-
Cholesteatoma 388-

Chondrocalcinosis, articular 279-
Chondrodysplasia 758-
Chondromalacia 739-
patellae 717-
Chorea
paralytic 355-
Sydenham's 390-
Choreo-athetosis 355-
Chromophytosis 110-
Cicatrix 709-
Circumcision, no disease V50-
Cirrhosis, liver (alcoholic) (portal) 571-
Claudication, intermittent 443-
Clawfoot
acquired 736-
congenital 754-
Cleft palate or lip 758-
Click, heart 7852
Climacteric female 627-
Clubfoot 754-
Clubhand 758-
Coagulation defects 287-
Coarctation aorta 746-
Coated tongue 528-
Coccidiomycosis 136-
Coccydynia 7242
Cold (common) 460-
COLD 492-
Colic
bilious 574-
infantile 7890
renal 7889
stools 574-
Colitis
allergic 558-
bacillary 008-
dietetic 558-
giardial 008-
infectious
presumed 009-
proven 008-
mucous 588-
regional 555-
spastic 558-
staphylococcal 008-
toxic 558-
ulcerative 555-
Collagen disease 725-
Collapsed lung 519-
Colospasm 558-
Colostomy V17-
Coma, diabetic 250-
Comedo 7061

Creeping eruption 127-
Cretinism 244-
Crohn's disease 555-
Croup 464-
asthmatic 493-
bronchial 466-
diphtheritic 136-
false 519-
Crush
syndrome 959-
with
   dislocation—*see* Dislocation
   fracture—*see* Fracture
   intact skin surface 929-
   internal organ injury 959-
   nerve injury 959-
   open wound—*see* Wound, open
Cryptitis 5646
Cryptorchism 7525
Crypt tonsil 463
Curvature of spine NOS 737-
Cushingoid 977-
correct substance, properly
   administered 279-
Cushing's syndrome 279-
Cut—*see* Wound, open
Cyanosis 7889
Cyclothymic personality 301-
Cyst
Baker's 7263
Bartholin's 629-
breast, benign 610-
bronchial 519-
cerebellum 355-
cervix uteri 629-
ear 7062
epidermoid 7062
mouth or oral soft tissue 528-
epithelial 7062
eye 378
follicular 629-
implantation dermoid 709-
   iris 378-
   mouth 528-
   vagina or vulva 629-
inclusion dermoid 7062
kidney 758-
knee (semilunar cartilage) 717-
lip 528-
Meibomian, infected 3730
ovary 629-
penis 607-
periodontal 520-

pilonidal 685-
popliteal 758-
rectal 579-
renal 758-
sebaceous 7062
synovial 7263
thyroglossal duct 758-
vaginal 629-
Cystic
disease of breast, chronic 610-
fibrosis 279-
Cystitis 595-
arising during pregnancy
   or puerperium 6466
Cystocele 618-
Cystostomy V10-
Cytology examination V70-

Dacryocystitis 378-
Dandruff 690-
Darier's disease 758-
Darwin's tubercle 758-
Deafness (acoustic) (complete)
   (conduction) (partial) 387-
noise induced 388-
traumatic 959-
word 7889
   developmental 315-
Death, unknown or
   undetermined cause 7889
Debility 7807
Decompression sickness 994-
Defect, congenital–*see*
   746- through 758-
Deficiency
ascorbic acid 260.
estrogen 279-
folic acid 260-
lipoprotein, familial 272-
niacin 260-
nutritional 260-
thiamin 260-
vitamin 260-
Deformity
acquired NEC 739-
alimentary tract, congenital 758-
ankle
   acquired NEC 736
     abduction, adduction,
     contraction, extension,
     flexion or rotation 739-
   congenital 758-
arm

Deformity, wrist (*cont.*)
  abduction, adduction,
    contraction, extension,
      flexion, or rotation 739-
  congenital 758-
Degeneration, degenerative
cerebellum 355-
cervical spine 723-
intervertebral disk (IV disk) 739-
lumbar (lumbosacral) 7244
thoracic spine 7244
Dehydration 279-
Delayed speech 7845
psychogenic 316-
Delay in development (physiological) 7834
mental 315-
Delinquency 312-
Delirium tremens 3031
Delivery (obstetrical)
with
  complication, any 661-
  fetopelvic disproportion 661-
  malpresentation 661-
  postpartum hemorrhage 661-
    delayed 661-
  premature delivery 6441
    outside of hospital V999
    baby V70-
without complication normal 650-
Delusions 295-
Dementia NOS 298-
senile (presenile) 294-
Dengue 136-
Dental
Abnormalities 520-
caries or cysts 520-
Dependent on drugs 3048
Depression NOS 3004
anxiety 3004
endogenous 296-
manic 296-
neurotic 3004
psychotic 296-
reactive 3004
  psychotic 296-
senile 294-
De Quervain's disease 7263
Derangement, knee 717-
acute, current injury 836-
chronic 717-
recurrent 739
Dermatitis NOS 692-
actinic (sunburn) 692-

allergic 692-
atopic 6918
contact 692-
diaper 6910
due to
  adhesive plaster or tape 692-
  caterpillar 692-
  cosmetic 692-
  drug applied to skin 692-
  poison ivy 692-
  sunlight 692-
  weather, cold or hot 692-
exfoliative (neonatorum) 709-
factitial 698-
flexural 6918
herpetiformis 709-
hypostatic, lower extremities 454-
infectious eczematoid 690-
medicamentosa, applied to skin 692-
nummular 692-
pruritic 692-
purulent 685-
radiation (radium) (roentgen)
    (x-ray) 692-
Rhus 692-
seborrhoeic 690-
septic 685-
stasis 454-
suppurative 685-
vegetans 685-
Dermatofibroma 216-
Dermatographia 708-
Dermatomycosis 110-
Dermatomyositis 725-
Dermatophytosis 110-
Dermatosis
erythematosquamous 690-
papulos nigra 709-
precancerous 709-
progressive pigmentary 709-
subcorneal 709-
Desmoid tumor 239-
Desquamation 685-
Destruction of eardrum 388-
Detached retina 378-
Development
lack of physiologic 7834
slow 7834
Deviation, deviated
septum 519-
sexual 316-
Diabetes NOS 250-
chemical (clinical) 7902

Dysentery, infectious (*cont.*)
  presumed 009-
  proven 008-
Dysesthesia 7820
Dysfunction
brain 355-
hepatic 571-
ventricular 429-
Dysgraphia 7889
Dyshidrosis 705-
Dyskeratosis 709-
Dysmenorrhea 6253
Dysostosis cleidocranial 758-
Dyspareunia NOS 6250
male 607-
psychogenic 3027
Dyspepsia 536-
Dysphagia 7889
Dysplasia
acetabular 754
cervical 622-
hip, congenital 758-
mammary, benign 610-
Dyspnea 7860
Dysuria 7881

Earache 388-
Ecchymosis NOS 459-
conjunctiva, spontaneous 378-
eye (eyelid), traumatic 929-
Eclampsia arising during pregnancy
        childbirth or puerperium 642-
Ecthyma 685-
Ectopic
heartbeat ('nodal') 4276
pregnancy 633-
Ectropion
cervix 622-
eyelid 378-
Eczema NOS 692-
atopic 6918
external auditory meatus 3801
infantile 6918
marginatum 136-
seborrhoeic 690-
  infantile 6918
vaccination (vaccinatum) 998-
Edema NOS 7823
allergic 9950
angioneurotic 9950
due to antifertility pill 9952
essential, acute 9950
hands 7823

legs NOS 7823
  due to obstruction 459-
pulmonary 519-
Edentulous 520-
Effects, adverse, of
chemicals, chiefly nonmedicinal 989-
complications of
  medical care 998-
  surgery 998-
medicinal agents 9952
  overdose or wrong substance 977-
physical agents (cold) (drowning)
        (heat) (lightning) 994-
sunlight 692-
Effort syndrome 3001
Effusion of
joint (chronic) 7190-
pleura NOS 5119
  serofibrinous 5119
  tuberculous 011-
Elephantiasis 459-
filiarial 127-
Elevated
blood
  chemistry finding NEC 7902
  pressure without
        diagnosis of hypertension 7962
hematologic finding NEC 2896
sedimentation rate 7900
urine test finding NEC 791-
Embolic CNS episode 355
Embolism 443-
artery 443-
cerebral 438-
kidney 598-
multiple 443-
paradoxical 443-
pulmonary 415-
Emesis 787-
complicating pregnancy 648-
Emotional
instability 301-
upset 300 9
Emphysema, pulmonary 492
Empty sella syndrome 279-
Empyema 519-
Encephalitis NOS 355-
epidemic (sleeping sickness) 136-
equine 136-
herpes (simplex virus) 054-
lead 989-
Murray Valley (Australian) 136-
postinfective 136-

Escape heartbeat 4276
Esophagitis 530-
Esophoria 378-
Esotropia 378-
Ethmoiditis 461-
Eustachian tube discomfort 388-
Eventration, diaphragm 758-
Examination
complete or partial V70-
cytology (Pap smear) V70-
health screening V70-
medical, with no disease detected V70-
newborn (well baby) V70-
postpartum V24-
prenatal V220
pre-operative V70-
to rule out or exclude specific disease V70-
X-ray V70-
Exanthem, viral NEC 057-
Exanthema subitum 057-
Excessive sweating 7808-
Excoriation
due to injury 918-
neurotic 698-
Exhaustion 7807
Exophthalmos NOS 378-
thyroid 242-
Exostosis 7263
Exotropia 378-
Exposure (to)
chemical(s) 989-
disease V01-
Extrasystoles 4276
Eye problems 378-

Failure
heart, right or left sided 428-
to thrive, in prenatal period 7834
renal 598-
respiratory 7889
ventricular, left 428-
Faint 7802
Family history of disease V10-
Family planning—*see* V251 through V256
Farmer's
lung 519-
skin 692-
Farsightedness 367-
Fasciculation 7810
Fasciitis, nodular 728-
Fatigue 7807
Favism 282-

Fear 3009
Fecal impaction 579-
Feeding problem in baby 7833
Felon 680-
Fertility, reduced 606-
Fever
cat-scratch 136-
from immunization 998-
glandular 075-
mosquito-borne 136-
relapsing 136-
rheumatic, acute 390-
scarlet 034-
unknown origin (FUO) 7806
Fibrillation
atrial (auricular) 4273
ventricular 429-
Fibro-adenosis, breast 610-
Fibrocystic breast 610-
Fibroid uterus 218-
Fibroma
prostate 600-
skin 216-
uterus 218-
Fibroplasia, retrolental 378-
Fibrosacroma 199-
Fibrosis
cystic 279-
pulmonary 519-
Fibrositis
shoulder 7260
site, other NEC 728-
Fifth disease 057-
Fill out forms V680
Fissure
anal 565-
nipple 611-
Fistula
anorectal 565-
cutaneous 685-
female genital tract 629-
pilonidal 685-
postoperative, persistent 998-
rectovaginal 629-
urethrovaginal 629-
Fixation, joint 739-
Flatfoot 736-
Flatulence 7873
Flexion contracture NEC 739-
Floater 378-
Floating
ribs 758-
testes 607-

Gallbladder disease 574-
Gallop rhythm of heart 429-
Gallstones 574-
Ganglion (of)
ankle 7274
joint 7274
knee 7274
popliteal space 7274
tendon sheath 7274
wrist 7274
Ganglioneuroma
benign 229-
malignant 199-
Gangrene 7889
gas (bacillus) 136-
Gas 7873
Gastritis (atrophic) (regional) 536-
acute 536-
Gastroenteritis NOS 009-
allergic 558-
dietetic 558-
dysentery (viral), presumed infectious 009-
infectious
presumed 009-
proven 008-
noninfectious 558-
toxic 558-
Genu
recurvatum 736-
congenital 754-
late effect of rickets 260-
valgum (knock knee) or
varum (bowlegs) 736-
congenital 758-
Geographic tongue 528-
Giardiasis 008-
Giddiness 7804
Gilbert's disease 279-
Gilles de la Tourette's disease 316-
Gingivitis 520-
Vincent's 136-
Gingivostomatitis 520-
herpetic 054-
Glaucoma 365-
Globus 3001
Glomerulonephritis, acute,
chronic, or subacute 580-
Glomerulosclerosis 578-
Kimmelstiel–Wilson 250- and 580-
Glossitis 528-
Glossodynia 528-
Glue
ear 3811

sniffing (addiction) 3048
Goiter
diffuse 240-
endemic 240-
nodular 242-
nontoxic 240-
nonendemic 240-
simple 240-
substernal 240-
toxic 242-
Gonococcal infection 098-
Gonorrhea 098-
Gout 274-
Grand mal 345-
Granuloma
annulare (lichen) 709-
facial 459-
inguinale 136-
liver 571-
monilial 112-
pyogenic 685-
silica, skin 709-
swimming pool 136-
urogenital 1121
Granulomatosis, Wegener's 459-
Grave's disease 242-
Green stools 7889
Grief reaction 308-
Gumma, syphilitic 090-
Gynecomastia 611-

Habitual drug abuse 3048
Halitosis 7889
Hallucination 7889
Hallucinosis 298-
alcoholic 3031
Hallux 736-
rigidus or valgus 736-
congenital 758-
Hammer toe 736-
congenital 758-
late effect of rickets 260-
Harelip 758-
Hay fever 477-
Headache NOS 7840
migraine 346-
sinus 461-
tension 3078
Heartbeat
awareness of 7851
ectopic 4276
escaped 4276

Hives 708-
Hoarseness 7845
Hodgkin's disease 201
Holding breath 312-
Hollow back 737-
Homesick 308-
Homosexuality 316-
Hordeolum 3730
Horn, cutaneous 709-
Horner's syndrome 355-
Hot flashes 627-
Hydatidiform mole 648-
Hydradenitis 705-
Hydrarthrosis (intermittent) 7190
Hydrocele (acquired) (congenital) 603-
Hydrocephalus
acquired 355-
congenital 758-
Hydronephrosis 598-
Hydrosalpinx 614-
Hygroma 228-
Hymen, imperforated 758-
Hyperactive
airway disease 519-
child 312-
Hyperaldosternonism 279-
Hyperalgesia 7820
Hyperalimentation 7889
vitamins 279-
Hyperbilirubinemia 279-
newborn 778-
Hypercalcemia 279-
Hypercholesterolemia 272-
Hyperesthesia(e) 7820
Hyperfunction of pituitary 279-
Hypergammaglobulinemia 2899
Hyperglycemia 7906
Hyperhydrosis 7808
Hyperinsulinism 279-
Hyperkalemia 279-
Hyperkeratosis 709-
Hyperkinesia, hyperkinetic
child 312-
heart syndrome 429-
Hyperlipemia 272-
Hyperlipidosis 272-
Hyperlipoproteinemia 272-
Hypermenorrhea 6262
Hypermobility, bowel 558-
Hyperopia 367-
Hyperparathyroidism 279-
Hyperpiesis 7962
Hyperpigmentation 709-

Hyperplasia, hyperplastic
adrenal 279-
cervix 622-
endometrium 629-
kidney 758-
prostatic 600-
Hyperproteinemia 279-
Hyperpyrexia 7806
Hypersplenism 2899
Hypertension, hypertensive 401-
benign 401-
causing
heart failure (congestive) 402-
hypertrophy, heart 402-
complications, with
pregnancy, childbirth or the puerperium 642-
renal sclerosis NOS or failure (chronic) 402-
encephalopathy 402-
essential 401-
heart disease 402-
labile (intermittent) 401-
lesser circulation 416-
malignant 402-
pulmonary 416-
primary 401-
secondary (to) (underlying cause)
aldosteronism 401- and 279-
diabetes 401- and 250-
renal involvement 402-
Hyperthyroidism 242-
Hypertrichosis 704-
Hypertriglyceridemia 272-
Hypertrophy
breast 611-
prostate, benign 600-
tonsils and/or adenoids 474-
Hyperuricemia 7902-
Hyperventilation syndrome 3001
Hypoalbuminemia 279-
Hypochondriasis 3001
Hypofunction of pituitary 279-
Hypoglycemia 279-
Hypogonadism 279-
Hypokalemia 279-
Hypomania 296-
Hypomenorrhea 6260
Hypoparathyroidism 279-
Hypopituitarism 279-
Hypospadias 758-
Hypotension
orthostatic 4580
postural 4580
Hypothyroidism 244-

Hypotonia, hypotony
bladder 598-
muscle 728-
Hysteria 3001

Illegitimacy V616
Ileus 579-
Illiterate V629
Immersion 994-
foot or hand 994-
Immunization, prophylactic V03-
Impaction
dental 520-
fecal 579-
fracture—*see* Fracture
intestine (calculous) (fecal) (gallstone)
    579-
Impetigo 684-
Impotence (psychogenic) (sexual) 3027
organic cause 607-
Inadequate personality 301-
Incompetent cervix 622-
in pregnancy 661-
Incontinence 7883
bowels 7889
fecal 7889
stress (female) 618-
    male 7883
urinary 7883
Increased
intracranial pressure 355-
Indigestion 536-
Infarction
myocardial 410-
postmyocardial 412-
pre-infarction, myocardial 410-
pulmonary 415-
subendocardial 410-
Infection
ear 3801
genital tract, arising during pregnancy
    670-
kidney NOS 5901
meningococcal 136-
mouth 528-
nail 680-
nose 519-
penis 607-
rectum 579-
sinus, pilonidal 685-
skin 685-
staphylococcal 136-
tearduct 378-

toe 685-
umbilical 685-
    newborn 778-
urinary tract NOS 595-
    arising during pregnancy or
        puerperium 6466
vaginal 6161
viral, unspecified 0799
wound 959-
Infertility
female 606-
male 606-
Infestation
filarial 127-
helminths 127-
larvae 132-
leeches 132-
maggots 132-
mites 133-
pinworms 127-
ringworm 110-
sand fleas 132-
Strongyloides stercoralis 127-
tinea 110-
Infiltrate
chest or lung 519-
Inflamed, inflammation
lung 486-
skin 685-
Influenza 487-
gastric 009-
Ingested
foreign
    body 930-
    substance 989-
Ingrown
hair 704-
toenail 703-
Inhailment environmental risk 989-
Injury
blast, with internal injury 959-
crushing 929-
    internal injury 959-
eardrum 959-
    perforation 889-
internal 959-
    abdomen, chest, or pelvis 959-
intracranial 850-
    with skull fracture 802-
teeth 889-
wound, open (laceration) 889-
Inoculation, prophylactic V03
Insomnia 7889

Insomnia (*cont.*)
nonorganic origin 3074
Instability
ankle 739-
personality 301-
Instruction, health V654-
education program V654-
Insufficiency, insufficient
cardiac 428-
cerebrovascular 438-
coronary 410-
dietary 260-
food (nourishment) 994-
   due to economic problem-
   add code V602
mental 317-
myocardial 428-
  with
      hypertension—*see* Hypertension
      rheumatic fever 390-
pancreatic 579-
pulmonary 519-
respiratory 7860
  in newborn 778-
valve, aortic or mitral 424-
  rheumatic 390-
vascular 459-
venous 454-
Intertrigo 709-
Intervertebral disc (disk) (degenerative)
     (prolapsed) (ruptured)
cervical 723-
lumbar (lumbosacral) 7244
thoracic 7244
Intestinal disease
infectious
  presumed 009-
  proven 008-
In-toeing 736-
Intolerance
food 579-
lactose 279-
Intoxication, alcohol
acute 3050
chronic 3031
Intussusception 579-
Inversion
foot 736-
nipple 611-
  puerperal 676-
Involuntary movements, abnormal 7819
Iritis 378-
Irregular

bowels 579-
menses 6262
pulse 429-
Irritable colon or bowel syndrome 558-
Irritation
bladder 598-
cervical 622-
eye 378-
nervous 7889
nose 519-
rectal 579-
vagina 629-
Ischemia, ischemic
attack, transient 435-
heart disease
  asymptomatic 412-
  chronic 412-
  subacute 410-
leg, Volkmann's (with peroneal nerve injury)
  959-
peripheral vascular condition 443-
  due to ergot ingestion-code also 977-
Itch NOS 698-
barbers' 110-
eye(s) 378-
filarial 127-
grain 133-
groin 110-
grocers' 133-
harvest 133-
rectal 698-
seven-year V611
  meaning acariasis, scabies or chiggers 133-
swimmers' 127-
vaginal 698-
washerwomen's 692-
water 127-
winter 698-

Jacksonian seizure (epilepsy) 345-
Jaundice NOS 7889
acholuric 282-
epidemic 070-
  leptospiral or spirochetal 136-
from injection, inoculation, or
transfusion 070-
hemolytic 285-
infectious 070-
obstructive 574-
Jealousy 312-
Jerks, myoclonic 355-

Keloid 709-

Lesion (*cont.*)
nose 519-
penis 607-
pulmonary NOS 579-
skin (pigmented) NOS 709-
vagina 629-
Lethargy 7807
Letters regarding patients V680
Leukocytosis 288-
Leukemia 201-
Leukopenia 2889
Leukoplakia 709-
cervix 622-
general 709-
oral 528-
penis 607-
tongue 528-
vagina 629-
Leukorrhea (fluor albus) 629-
Lice 132-
Lichen NOS 709-
myxedematous 709-
nitidus 709-
planus 709-
sclerosis et atrophicus 709-
simplex, chronic 698-
Light headedness 7804
Lipoma 214-
Lithiasis, renal 592-
Liver disease 571-
Locking of joint 739-
knee 717-
Loose
bodies, joint 739-
  knee 717-
Lordosis
acquired 737-
congenital 758-
tuberculous 011-
Loss of
appetite 7830
hair 704-
hearing 387-
libido 3027
memory 7889
smell 7889
taste 7889
touch 7820
weight 7832
Low
blood pressure 4580
hemoglobin 285-
IQ 317-

Low-output syndrome 429-
Lumbago 7242
Lumbar disc disease 739-
Lupus
erythematosis
  discoid (chronic) 709-
  local 709
  systemic (disseminated) 725-
vulgaris 011-
Lymphadenitis NOS 2891
acute 683-
chronic 2891
mesenteric 2891
Lymphadenopathy NOS 7856
Lymphangioma (simple) 228-
malignant 199-
Lymphangitis (lymphangiitis) 459-
Lymphedema
acquired (chronic) (secondary) 459-
hereditary (Milroy's disease) 459-
postoperative 998-
  postmastectomy 459-
primary (praecox) 459-
Lymphocytosis 288-
acute, infectious 075-
Lymphogranuloma
malignant 201-
venereal (inguinale) 136-
Lymphoma 201-
Burkitt's 201-
following renal transplant 201- and V10-
leukemic 201-
malignant (Hodgkin's) (lymphosarcoma) 201-

Maggots 132
Malabsorption syndrome 579-
Maladjustment—*see also* Problem(s)
adolescent—*see* V612 and 308-
marital—*see* V611 and 308-
occupation V620
school V623
social V624
Malaise 7807
Malaria 084-
Malingering V670
Mallett finger 736-
Mallow–Weiss tear 530-
Malnutrition NOS 260-
baby 260-
  due to neglect 9950
intra-uterine 778-
kwashiorkor 260-
protein 260-

Milroy's disease 758-
Miosis 373-
Miscarriage 634-
Mites 133-
Mitral
insufficiency 424-
 rheumatic 390-
regurgitation 424-
 rheumatic 390-
stenosis 390-
 nonrheumatic 424-
Mittelschmerz 6253
Mole
benign 216-
hydatidiform 648-
malignant 173-
Molested 959-
Molluscum contagiosum (water wart) 136-
Mongolian, mongolism, mongoloid 758-
spot 758-
Monilia, moniliasis 112-
urogenital site 1121
Mononucleosis, infectious 075-
Morton's toe (foot) (neuroma) 355-
Motion sickness 994-
Mountain sickness (altitude) 994-
Mucocele, salivary gland 528-
Multiple sclerosis 340-
Mumps (orchitis) 072-
Munchausen syndrome 301-
Murmur, heart (functional) (innocent) 7852
mitral stenotic 390
 nonrheumatic 424-
systolic 424-
Muscle
cramp 7295
 due to immersion 994-
 leg 7295
pull—*see* Sprain
spasm
 due to sprain or strain—*see* Sprain
 involuntary movements, abnormal 7810
Muscular dystrophy 355-
Myalgia 728-
epidemic 136-
Myasthenia gravis 355-
Myelitis 355-
Myeloma (benign) (multiple) 201-
Myelopathy 355-
cervical 721-
lumbar (lumbosacral) 721-
thoracic 721-
Myiasis 132-

Myocardial infarction 410-
postmyocardial infarct (healed) 412-
Myocardiopathy, idiopathic 429-
Myocarditis (chronic) 429-
rheumatic 390-
Myeloproliferative syndrome 239-
Myofascitis 728-
Myoma, uterus 218-
Myopathy 355-
Myopia 367-
Myositis NOS 728-
fibrosis 728-
 Volkmann's contracture 959-
Myringitis 388-
traumatic 889-
Myxedema (circumscribed) 244-

Narcolepsy 355-
Nasal stuffiness 7889
Nasopharyngitis 460-
Nausea with or without vomiting 7870
Near drowning 994-
Nearsightedness (myopia) 367-
Necrosis
fat 728-
 breast 611-
hip 739-
Neoplasm
benign
 breast 217-
 gastrointestinal tract 229-
 hemangioma 227-
 lipoma 214-
 lymphangioma 228-
 site, other NEC 229-
 skin 216-
 uterus (cervix uteri) 218-
in-situ 199-
 cervix 180-
malignant
 adnexa 199-
 anus 151-
 basal cell 173-
 bladder 188-
 breast 174-
 bronchus 162-
 cervix 180
 colon 151-
 endometrium 180-
 epiglottis 162-
 esophagus 151-
 face 199-
 squamous cell 173-

Nosebleed 7847
Numbness 7820
Nursing home transfer V999
Nutrition, poor 260-
due to insufficient food 994-

Obesity 278-
Observation (of)
high-risk patient
 implants or transplants V10-
 medication V14-
 prosthetic implants V10-
without need for further medical
  care at this time V70-
Obstruction, obstructive
esophagus 530-
eustachian 3815
intestinal (bowel) (colon) 579-
prostatic 600-
pulmonary (lung) disease 492-
Occlusion, occluded
aorto-iliac 443-
tear duct 378-
 congenital 7436
Oesophagitis 530-
Oligomenorrhea 6260-
Oligospermia 606-
Omphalitis 685-
Onychogryphosis 703-
Onychomycosis 110-
Onychorrhexis (brittle nails) 703-
Onychotrophia (atrophy) 703-
Oophoritis
acute or chronic 614-
gonococcal 098-
Opacification
corneal 378-
Ophthalmia NOS 3720
allergic 3720
 with hay fever 477-
gonococcal 098-
migraine 346-
nodosa 378-
sympathetic 378-
Oral contraception—*see* V255
Orchialgia 607-
Orchitis NOS 604-
gonococcal 098-
mumps 072-
nonspecific 604-
septic 604-
suppurative 604-
syphilitic 090-

tuberculous 011-
Organic
brain syndrome 316-
heart disease 429-
Orthopnea 7860
Orthostatic
albuminuria 5936
proteinuria 5936
Osgood–Schlatter's disease 732-
Osteitis NOS 739-
deformans 739-
jaw 520-
Osteoarthritis, osteoarthrosis 715-
deformans alkaptonurica 279-
spine 721-
Osteoarthropathy 715-
hypertrophic secondary (pulmonary) 715-
Osteochondritis
dissecans 732-
metatarsal (head) 732-
vertebral 732-
Osteochondroma 229-
Osteochondromatosis 239-
synovial 7263
Osteochondrosis 732-
Osteogenesis imperfecta 758-
Osteoma 229-
Osteomalacia 260-
Osteomyelitis NOS 739-
chronic 739-
focal 739-
sclerosing 739-
suppurative 739-
Osteoporosis 7330
postmenopausal 7330
post-traumatic 739-
senile 7330
Osteosarcoma 199-
Otalgia 388-
Otitis NOS 3820
acute
 secretory (nonsuppurative) 3811
 suppurative 3820
chronic 3820
externa 3801
 tropical 110-
exudative, chronic 3811
nonsuppurative 3811
serous, chronic 3811
suppurative 3820
 chronic 388-
unspecified 3820
with mastoiditis—*code both*

Palpitations 7851
Palsy NOS 355-
Bell's 355-
cerebral 355-
shaking 332-
Pancreatitis 579-
acute or chronic 579-
Panniculitis 728-
Pansinusitis 461-
Pap smear
negative V70-
performed V70-
suspicious, not yet diagnosed 7950
Papilledema 378-
Papilloma
mouth 228-
uterus 218-
Papule 709-
Paralysis
agitans (Parkinsonism) 332-
facial 355-
familial periodic 355-
nerve 355-
post-stroke 438-
progressive bulbar 355-
spastic 355-
Paranoia 295-
Paranoid personality 301-
Parapertussis 033-
Paraphasia 7845
Paraphimosis 605-
Paraplegia 355-
Parapsoriasis 709-
Parascarlatina 057-
Parasites, intestinal 127-
Parasystole, ventricular 4276
Paratyphoid 008-
carrier V01-
Paresis
general 090-
unspecified 355-
Paresthesia 7820
Parkinsonism 332-
idiopathic (disease) 332-
syndrome (postencephalitic)
        (symptomatic) 332-
Paronychia 680-
Parotitis 528-
epidemic (mumps) 072-
not mumps 528-
postoperative 528-
Patches
mucous 090-

smokers' 528-
Pectus carinatum or excavatum
acquired 739-
congenital 758-
Pediculosis, all sites 132-
Pellegrini-Stieda disease 7263
Pellagra 260-
Pemphigus, pemphigoid 709-
neonatorum (impetigo) 684-
Peptic ulcer 533-
Perforated, perforation
by
    foreign body (object) (in)
        eardrum 889-
        entering through orifice (mouth)
            rectum 939-
        eye (adnexa) 930-
        skin laceration or puncture 889-
            superficial 912-
    intra-uterine device (IUD) 998-
intestine
    due to internal injury 959-
    nontraumatic 579-
    obstetric trauma 661-
surgical, accidental 998-
tympanum 388
    traumatic 889-
with foreign body in tissue 889-
    superficial 912-
Peri-arthritis 7263
shoulder 7260
Pericapsulitis, adhesive 7260
Percarditis 429-
rheumatic (fever) 390-
viral 429-
Pericystitis 595-
Perihepatitis 571-
Perilabyrinthitis 386-
Perinephritis 5901
purulent 598-
Periodic
edema 9950
fever 279-
paralysis 355-
peritonitis 279-
Periodontitis 520-
Periodontosis 520-
Peri-oophoritis 614-
Periostitis 739-
Periphlebitis 451-
Perisalpingitis 614-
Peritendinitis 7263
shoulder 7260

Plummer-Vinson syndrome (anemia) 280-
Pneumatocele 519-
Pneumoconiosis 519-
Pneumomediastinum 519-
Pneumonia NOS 486-
aspiration 519-
bacterial 486-
cold agglutinin positive 486-
Eaton agent 486-
eosinophylic, chronic 519-
influenzal 486-
irradiation 519-
Klebsiella 486-
lipid 519-
lobar 486-
newborn (aspiration) 778-
pneumococcal 486-
primary atypical 486-
staphylococcal 486-
viral 486-
Pneumonitis, allergic 519-
Pneumopericardium 429-
Pneumothorax, spontaneous 519-
Podagra 274-
Poison ivy or oak 692-
Poisoning (by)
Bacillus 008-
bacterial toxins 008-
blood—see Septicemia
botulism 008-
chemicals or drugs
    medicinal 977-
    nonmedicinal, chiefly 989-
fava bean 282-
food (fish) (meat) (Salmonella)
    (Staphylococcus) 008-
    bacterial 008-
    infected 008-
    noxious foodstuffs such as
        mushrooms 989-
lead 989-
medicinal drugs 977-
nonmedicinal chemicals 989-
pork infested with trichinosis 127-
shellfish, noxious 989-
uric acid 274-
Polioencephalomyelitis 045-
Polioencephalopathy 260-
Poliomyelitis (abortive) (nonparalytic)
    (paralytic) (late effects) 045-
chronic 355-
contact with suspected or proven carrier
    V01-

Polyarteritis nodosa 459-
Polyarthralgia 7194
psychogenic 3001
Polyarthritis 725-
Polycystic kidney 758-
Polycythemia 239-
acquired 2899
benign 2899
secondary 2899
Polydipsia 7889
Polymenorrhea 6262
Polymyalgia rheumatica 725-
Polymyositis 725-
Polyneuritis 355-
Polyneuropathy 355-
due to lead or arsenic 989-
Polyp
adenomatous 216-
    of cervix 218-
cervical 622-
    in pregnancy or childbirth 661-
colon 229-
dental 520-
ear 388-
larynx 519-
middle ear 388-
nose 519-
rectum 579-
sinus 519-
skin 709-
urethral 598-
vagina 629-
vocal cords 519-
Polyphagia 7889
Polyposis 229-
Polyuria 7884
Pompholyx (dyshidrosis) 705-
Porphyria NOS 279-
associated with drug addiction 3048
due to drugs (medicinal) 9952
    overdose or wrong substance 977-
secondary 279-
Postcardiotomy syndrome 429-
Postmastectomy syndrome 459-
Postmaturity syndrome 778-
Postmyocardial infarction syndrome 412-
Post nasal drip 460-
Postnatal care V70-
Postpartum care V24
Post-stroke paralysis 438-
Preauricular sinus tract 758-
Presbyacusis 386-
Pre-eclampsia 642-

Problems, legal (*cont.*)
  imprisonment V625
  insurance settlement V625
  juvenile delinquency (court)—*see*
    312- and V623 or V625
  legal investigations V625
  litigation V625
    divorce V610
  nonpayment of child support V602
  separation V610
 living alone
  loneliness V624
    grief reaction 308-
  need for housekeeper or
    nursing aide V629
 marital V611
  sexual activity *see* 3027 or 316-
 medical care of sick person V614
 occupational V620
  difficulty holding job V620
  dissatisfaction with present job V620
  frustration in selecting career V620
  unemployment V620
 offspring unwilling or unable to
    care for sick parent V614
 other, not classifiable to 008- through V629,
  V999
 parent-child
  adopted or foster child V612
  battered child see V612 and 9950
  behavior of child V612
  child
    abuse V612 or 9950
    affected by discord
      between parents V610
    neglect V612
    suspected or known to be
      drug or alcohol abuser V612
 phase of life V627
  aging process V627
 pregnancy out of wedlock V616
 responsibility
  no one to care for sick patient V614
  of patient for relative(s) V651
  spouse unable to take care of mate V614
 Social
  adjustment NEC V629
  maladjustment V624
    grief caused by death in family 308-
 transportation
  distance too great V999
  economic difficulty V602
Procidentia uteri 618-

Proctalgia fugax 5646
Proctitis 5646
Prolapse, prolapsed
disc (disk)
  cervical 723-
  lumbar (lumbosacral) 7244
  thoracic 7244
uterovaginal 618-
Prolonged gestation syndrome 778-
Pronation, foot 736-
congenital 758-
Prostatism 600-
Prostatitis 600-
acute or chronic 601-
trichomonal 1310
Prosthetic device requiring close
    observation and care V10-
Proteinuria 791-
Protozoal intestinal disease,
    proven 008-
Prurigo 698-
Pruritis (ani) (anogenital) 698-
Pseudo-arthrosis 739-
Pseudocyesis (false pregnancy) 3001
Pseudogout syndrome 279-
Pseudohermaphroditism 758-
endocrine disorder 279-
Pseudopsoriasis 6961
Pseudoscarlatina 057-
Pseudotumor cerebri 355-
Pseudoxanthoma elasticum 758-
Psittacosis 136-
Psoriasis (pustular) (with or without arthropathy)
  6961
Psychalgia 3078
Psychogenic
air hunger 3001
asthma 3001
cardiovascular disorder 3001
cough 3001
heart rhythm or disease 3001
hyperventilation 3001
yawning 3001
Psychophysiologic disorder
urogenital system
Psychosis NOS 298-
affective 296-
alcoholic 3031
brain syndrome 294-
depressive 296-
due to drug or chemical
    intoxication 3048
hysterical, acute 298-

Reaction (*cont.*)
depressive 3004
  affective 296-
  psychotic 298-
dissociative 3001
drug
  contact (skin) 692-
  external 692-
 · ingested
    correct substance 9950
    overdose or wrong substance 977-
grief 308-
group delinquency 312-
hypochondriacal 3001
insulin 9952
lumbar puncture 355-
neurotic 3009
obsessive (compulsion) 3009
overanxious, child or adolescent 312-
paranoid 295-
personality 301-
phobic 3009
runaway 312-
situational 308-
spinal puncture 355-
spite 312
stress, acute 308-
stress, chronic—*see* Problem(s)
tetanus-antitoxin 998-
toxin-antitoxin 998-
unsocialized 312-
withdrawing 312-
X-ray
  accidental 994-
  due to
    inadvertent exposure 994-
    therapy (medical care) 994-
Recklinghausen's (disease)
neurofibromatosis 239-
of bones 279-
Rectocele 618-
Red eye 378-
Reduced
libido 3027
visual acuity 369-
Redundant
foreskin 605-
skin (facial) 709-
  eyelids 378-
Referral of patient without need
    for examination or interview V683
Reflux
esophageal 530-

ureteral 598-
Refractive errors 367-
Regurgitation
aortic 424-
  rheumatic 390-
food 7870
Reiter's syndrome 136-
with arthritis—code also 725-
Relaxation, pelvic floor 618-
Renal
failure 598-
stone 592-
'Restless leg' syndrome 355-
Retardation
growth 7834
mental 317-
Retention, fluid 279-
Retinopathy, hypertensive—*see* Hypertension
Retraction, uterus 629-
Retrovision
femoral 754-
uterus 629-
Rhabdomyolysis 728-
Rh incompatibility (mother) 661-
Rheumatic
fever 390-
heart disease 390-
stenosis of aortic valve 390-
valvulitis 390-
Rheumatism, nonarticular
palindromic 725-
shoulder 7260
site, other NEC 728-
Rheumatoid
arthritis 714-
carditis 714-
Rhinitis NOS 519-
acute (common cold) 460-
allergic (nonseasonal) (seasonal) 477-
atopic 477-
atrophic (ozena) 519-
chronic (hyperplastic) (hypertrophic) 519-
vasomotor 477-
Rhinophyma 709-
Rhinorrhea 519-
allergic 477-
Rhythm
coronary sinus 429-
gallop 429-
sinus arrhythmia 429-
ventricular conduction, aberrant 429-
Rickets 260-
Ringing in ears 388-

Shock, anaphylactic (*cont.*)
  drugs (medications) 977-
   serum or inoculation 977-
 electric 994-
 following injury 959-
 insulin 279-
 lightning 994-
Short
 breath 7860
 hamstring 739-
 leg
  .acquired 736-
  congenital 754-
Shoulder-hand syndrome 355-
Sickle cell anemia or trait 282-
Sickness
 air travel 994-
 altitude 994-
 car 994-
 motion 994-
 sleeping 136-
 travel 994-
Sever's disease 732-
Sinus
 arrest 429-
 arrhythmia 429-
 pauses 429-
Sinusitis, acute or chronic 461-
Sixth disease 057-
Sjogren's syndrome 725-
Sleep
 disorder, psychogenic 3074
 walking 3074
Slipped disc (disk)
 cervical 723-
 lumbar (lumbosacral) 7242
 thoracic 7242
Slipping patella 717-
Slurred speech 7845
Small for age
 neo-natal period 778-
 adult 279-
Smallpox 136-
Smoker 3051
Smoker's mouth patches 528-
Snapping
 fingers (thumb) 7263
 jaw 520-
 knee 717-
Sniffles 460-
Snow blindness 378-
Soldier's heart 3001
Somnambulism 3074

Somnolence 3074
Sore
 nose 519-
 skin 709-
 throat 460-
  streptococcal 034-
 tongue 528-
Spasm NOS 7810
 anal 5646
 bladder 598-
 cervical 7810
 esophagus 530-
 habit (tic) 316-
 intestinal (anal) (colon) 558-
 muscle
  due to sprain or strain—*see* Sprain
  involuntary, abnormal 7810
 nervous 3001
 trigeminal nerve 355-
Speech
 disturbance 7845
 impediment NEC 7845
  psychogenic 316-
Spermatocele 607-
Spherocytosis 282-
Spina bifida 758-
Splenic flexure syndrome 579-
Splenomegaly 7891
Spondylitis NOS 7242
 ankylosing 714-
 osteo-arthritic 721-
 rheumatoid 714-
 tuberculous 011-
Spondylolisthesis, congenital 758-
Spondylosis
 cervical 721-
 degenerative 721-
 spinal (lumbar) 721-
Sporotrichosis 136-
Spots
 atrophic 709-
 cafe au lait 709-
 Mongolian (pigmented) 758-
Spotting, intermenstrual 6262
Sprain or strain (joint) (ligament) (muscle) (tendon)
 ankle 8450
 arm 840-
 back, except neck 840-
  low, chronic 728-
 carpal 842-
 cartilage
  costal 848-
  knee 844-

Trigger finger 7263
Trigonitis 595-
Truancy, childhood 312-
with education problem–code also V623
Tubercule, Darwin's 758-
Tuberculosis
all sites 011-
contact with V01-
late effects 011-
positive conversion test 011-
Tularemia 136-
Tussive syncope 7862
Tympanic membrane rupture
nontraumatic history 388-
traumatic 889-
Tympanitis 388-
Tympanosclerosis 388-
Typhoid 008-
carrier (state) V01-
Typhus (endemic (epidemic) 136-

Ulcer
aphthous, oral (stomatitis) 528-
cervix 622-
chronic, varicose, of leg 454-
corneal 378-
Curling's—*see* 532- and 533-
decubitus 707-
duodenal 532-
gastric 533-
gastrojejunal 533-
Hunner's 595-
hypertensive or ischemic, of legs 707-
   and code also the hypertension
lower extremity
   atrophic 707-
   chronic 707-
   decubitus 707-
   pyogenic 707-
   varicose 454-
marginal (anastomotic) (stomal) 533-
nose 519-
palate 528-
penis 607-
peptic 533-
pyloric 533-
rodent (skin) 173-
skin 707
stasis, varicose 454-
stomal (gastrojejunal) 533-
trophic, decubitus 707-
tropical 707-
varicose 454-

with gangrene—code also 7889
Underdevelopment, physiologic 7834
Underweight NOS 7834
due to
   feeding problem in baby 7833
   weight loss 7832
Undescended testicle 7525
Unmarried parenthood female V616
male V629
Unretractable foreskin 605-
Upper respiratory (tract) infection, acute 460-
Uremia 598-
Ureteral calculus 592-
Urethral calculus 592-
Urethritis
abacterial 597-
acute 597-
gonococcal (acute) 098-
nongonorrheal 597-
nonspecific (acute) 0994-
not sexually transmitted 597-
trichomonal 1310
Urethrocele 629-
URI 460-
Urine test, abnormal, not yet diagnosed 791-
Urticaria
allergic 708-
cholinergic 708-
giant (angioneurotic edema) 708-
nonallergic 708-
papular (lichen urticatus) 698-
pigmentosa 758-
Uterine retrodisplacement 629-

Vaccination
prophylactic V03-
reaction 998-
vaccinia (generalized reaction) 998-
Vaginal prolapse 618-
Vaginitis NOS 6161
gonococcal 098-
granuloma 136-
hemophilus vaginalis 6161
monilia 1121
mycotic 1121
nonspecific or atrophic 6161
senile (atrophic) 627-
trichomonal 1310
Vaginismus 6250
Valvulitis, heart 424-
atherosclerotic 424-
rheumatic 390-

Weak, weakness NOS 7807
joint 739-
limb 739-
muscle 728-
newborn 778-
senile 797-
Weather
effects of NEC 994-
skin 692-
Weight loss 7832
Well baby, care of examination V70-
Wen 7062
Wheal 709-
Wheezing 7860
'Whiplash' injury (neck) 8470
Whisper speech 7845
Whooping cough 033-
Withdrawal syndrome (drug) (narcotic) 3048
Wolf–Parkinson–White syndrome
paroxysmal tachycardia 4270
other 429-
Worms 127-
Wound
open (by firearms) (cutting) (ligament) (muscle)
(penetrating) (perforating) (tendon)
abdominal wall 889-
animal bite 889-
cerebral 850-
eye 889-
foot 889-
groin or flank 889-
hand 889-
head 889-
internal organ of abdomen, chest, or

pelvis (heart) (intestine)
(liver) (lungs) 959-
limb (lower) (upper) 889-
neck 889-
trunk 889-
internal organ 959-
with foreign body in tissue 889-
superficial 912-
superficial 918-
insect bite 910-
Wrinkling of facial skin 709-
Wrist drop 736-
Wry neck 723-
Wucheria infestation 127-

Xanthelasma 272-
Xeroderma 758-
Xerosis 709-
Xerostomia 528-
X-ray
abnormal findings, not yet diagnosed 793-
adverse effects of
due to
inadvertent exposure 994-
therapy complication 994-
industrial 994-
examination V70-

Yawning, psychogenic 3001
Yaws 136-

Zona 053-
Zoster 053-